MODERN DANCE: BODY AND MIND
A BASIC APPROACH FOR BEGINNERS

Sandra Cerny Minton, Ph.D.
with contributions by
Karen Genoff, M.Ed.
University of Northern Colorado,
Greeley, Colorado

Morton Publishing Company
295 W. Hampden, Suite 104
Englewood, Colorado 80110

DEDICATION

To my parents, Leona and William Cerny, who encouraged me to be interested and curious; to my friends for their continued support and encouragement; and to Dr. Alma Hawkins, who helped me dare to create.

Printed in the United States of America

ISBN: 0-89582-102-8

CONTENTS

ACKNOWLEDGMENTS

Special appreciation is given to the following individuals:

> Kay Carara, Gregory Gonzales, and Judy Hoffman, who posed for the photographs in this book; and

> Elizabeth Robb and Bradford Beckwith, who appear in the cover photo.

> The authors also wish to express their thanks to Dr. Cynthia Carlisle of the University of Northern Colorado for help in proofreading the text.

CREDITS

Illustrations by Susan Strawn

Text photographer Dr. James Bryant
Metropolitan State College, Denver

Cover photograph Centennial Photo/Bill Scherer of *Taking It In*
choreographed by Cynthia Howell

PREFACE

The desire in writing this book is to provide a basic approach to learning modern dance. The areas of technique, improvisation, and composition are described so that students can have a total picture of the subject matter included under the broad title of modern dance. In the first chapter, a brief summary outlines the work of the modern dance pioneers in order to provide an understanding of the origins of this dance form. Second, an effort has been made to talk about both the mental and physical aspects of dance movement. A discussion of the skeletal framework, the muscular system, different body types, nutrition, and dance injuries are included under the physical aspects of dancing. There has also been an attempt to name movements using anatomical terminology and descriptions. Chapter 3 includes a summary of the basic goals involved in most dance classes plus an analysis of positions and movements most likely to be found in the typical beginning modern dance experience.

The mental aspects of learning modern dance are discussed in Chapter 4. It is the wish that the suggestions provided in this chapter will help students perceive human motion in a way that will enable them to develop a framework in which to analyze and learn movements and movement combinations presented in class. Hopefully, this approach will cut down on the confusion often experienced by beginners. Additional suggestions for improving concentration and reducing tension are also included.

Many photographs and drawings have been provided throughout this book. These illustrations should be used to clarify written descriptions of movement — particularly when they are referred to in the text.

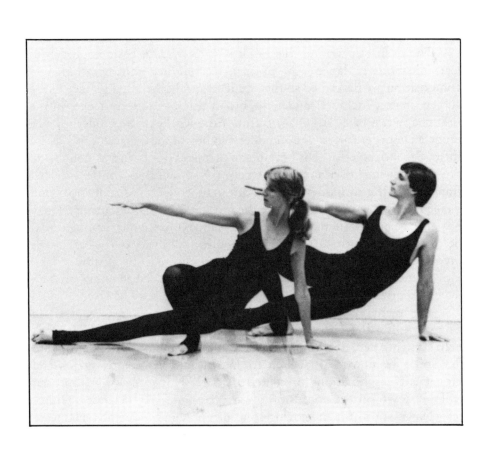

CHAPTER 1

An Introduction to Modern Dance

Dance has been enjoying an increased popularity for the last ten years, a popularity that is due in part to the prevalence of dance seen in films such as A *Turning Point, All That Jazz,* and *Flash Dance*; musical productions like *Dancin'* and A *Chorus Line*; and in television shows of the nature of *Fame.* The advent of aerobic exercise and aerobic dancing have also done much to interest the public in other dance forms, so that many people regularly participate in a jazz, modern dance, or ballet class in order to keep trim.

A well-planned dance class exercises all parts of the body, providing stretching, strengthening, and endurance activities at different points in the lesson. Dancing can wake you up and create an overall awareness of your body, leaving you with a feeling of general well-being and relaxation. Musical accompaniment used in a dance class adds to the fun and contributes to the motivational energy during class. Today, dancing can be a lifetime leisure activity, and it is being used increasingly as an exercise form for senior citizens.

What is Modern Dance?

Modern dance includes several areas of dance movement. First, it is a training system for the body called dance technique. Through dance technique, you learn how to control your body and make it your instrument. Technique provides the skills of dance movement, so that you can move efficiently and with precision.

Improvisation is a second area encompassed by the title modern dance. Improvisation refers to spontaneous movement performed by students in response to suggestions by the teacher. Motivations for improvisation can be various images, ideas, feelings, or other stimuli that cause you to relate and move. Furthermore, these images can be visual, verbal, auditory, kinesthetic, or even tactile in nature.

Improvisation can be done just for the fun of it, or it can result in a series of movements or phrases to be included in a dance composition, the third area of concern for the modern dancer. A composed or choreographed dance is arranged in a set form that can ideally be performed time and again in the same manner. It has a beginning, middle, and end and is made up of many phrases of movement that have been carefully placed in ordered sequences to formulate the whole. Sometimes the intent behind a choreography is to project a specific message to the audience. In such cases, the composition is structured so that it tells a story. In other instances, the choreographer's motivation is to experiment with movement to create a dance in a cohesive style without any story line as intent.

The philosophy behind modern dance allows considerable freedom to the dancer. This freedom can be found in both technique and in choreography. Modern dance, for example, has many different technical styles or training systems. Each has been invented by a well-known professional dancer who sought to devise his/her own method of providing dance students with movement skills. Each training system involves the same or similar dance goals such as flexibility, strength, and endurance but encompasses different sequences and series of movements. The different technical systems in modern dance are usually named after the professional dancer who created them, so that there are the techniques of Doris Humphrey, Martha Graham, Merce Cunningham, Erick Hawkins, and many others.

Choreographic freedom is also part of the philosophy behind modern dance. The choreographer needs to be clear concerning the motivation for a dance, but the intent and style of the choreography are not restricted to certain areas or subject matter. They are of the choreographer's own choosing.

Where Did Modern Dance Come From?

Modern dance arose at the beginning of the twentieth century through the efforts of a group of pioneering dancers. These dancers sought to create a movement form that was different from the already established ballet and that suited the tempo and pulse of the new century.

One of the first professional dancers to experiment with new and creative ideas was a woman named Loie Fuller, an American performer born in 1862. Fuller was first an actress and later a dancer. She lacked technical training but became known for her work with movement, material, and theatrical lighting effects. It has been said that Fuller stumbled upon her unusual dance form when she was onstage and realized the artistic potential of her billowing and gauzy skirt as she moved through the beams of light from the various lighting instruments.[1]

Electricity was one of the new inventions of the time, and Fuller capitalized on the magical effects that she was able to achieve by swirling her silk draperies and sheer skirts in front of these lights. She also experimented with phosphorescent radium paint on some of her costumes, creating a dancer bathed in an ethereal glow.[2]

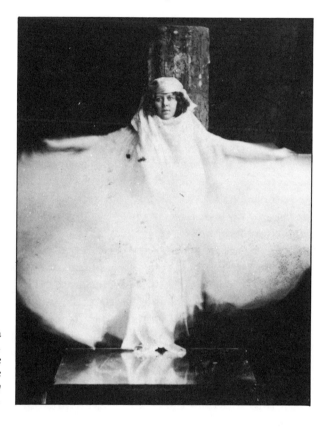

Loie Fuller, 1896, in an unidentified dance pose. Photograph courtesy of the Dance Collection, The New York Public Library at Lincoln Center.

Probably the most known and celebrated of the early modern dancers was Isadora Duncan. She was born in 1878 and grew up in San Francisco. Duncan loved to dance as a young girl but soon found that the then popular ballet did not suit her temperament and movement style. Instead, she sought to create her own dance forms that would allow her to express herself in motion. Duncan learned to dance from the center of the body, which she called the solar plexis or emotional center.[3] From this center, energy flowed outward, providing impulses for her actions. Those who saw Duncan perform said that her dancing appeared natural and so free-flowing that it looked like it was being created on the spot. In essence, her dancing was an unconventional and personal form of expression.[4] In contrast to Fuller, Duncan had less emphasis on theatrical effects and more interest in pure movement and the use of the body.

Another of Duncan's ideas was to recreate the classical ideals of the ancient Greeks through her dancing. Her favorite costume was a Grecian style tunic that she felt enhanced the classic simplicity of her movements.[5] The music for Isadora's dances were the great musical works of her time, many of which were impressive and powerful.

Isadora Duncan achieved her greatest popularity in Europe, particularly in France, Germany, and Russia, where she had dance schools and where her work influenced both ballet and modern dance choreography for many years.[6] In 1927, Isadora Duncan died in a tragic automobile accident in which she was choked to death when a long scarf that she was wearing became tangled around one of the axles of her car. Throughout her life, Duncan pursued her own unique path, so that her life, like her dancing, was free in spirit — often without regard for the traditional morals or ideals of the day.[7]

Ruth St. Denis, born in 1877, was another important pioneer of the modern dance. As a child in New Jersey, St. Denis loved to dance, and she studied ballet, social dancing, and the movement education system devised by Françoise Delsarte for training actors in expressive movement. Her choreographic career was inspired when she saw a picture of an ancient Egyptian goddess on a poster advertising cigarettes. Ruth St. Denis was determined to create a dance in which she was that Egyptian goddess. The dances that she created were called *The Cobras* and *Radha*, and they were performed at gentlemen'c "smokers."[8] These two works were the first of many eastern style dances composed by St. Denis in which she sought to project her impressions of the ethnic dance forms. Later in her career, Ruth St. Denis adopted other choreographic styles. Among these was her interest in large group dances, which she called music visualizations. In these choreographies, the individual dancers performed the note values and melody line of particular instruments in the musical score.[9]

In 1914, St. Denis married Ted Shawn, whom she met while touring the country. Ted Shawn, who had grown up in Denver, had first studied to be a minister. Ill health, however, forced Shawn to discontinue his religious studies, and as part of his physical therapy, he began dancing. St. Denis and Shawn formed Denishawn, a touring dance company that traveled throughout the United States extensively until 1932, performing in many different cities and on college campuses across the nation. Together, these two dancers did more than any of the other modern dance pioneers to bring the new dance forms to American people. Both dancers performed with the company and choreographed new works for it. Shawn, however, did more of the organizational work, while St. Denis was more the mystic and visionary of the two.[10] They also ran schools in Los Angeles and New York, where many of their young performers were

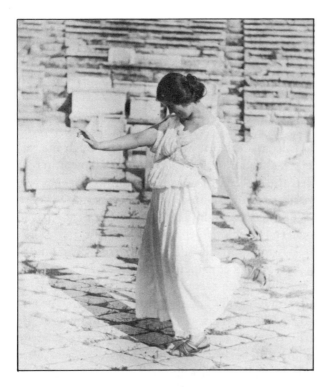

Isadora Duncan dancing
in an outdoor theater,
Athens, Greece, 1904.
Courtesy of the Dance
Collection, The New York
Public Library at Lincoln
Center.

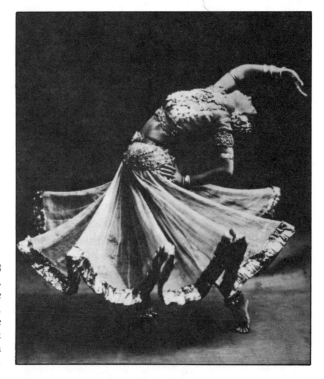

Ruth St. Denis 1906-08
dancing **Radha.**
Photograph from the
Denishawn Collection,
courtesy of the Dance
Collection, The New York
Public Library at Lincoln
Center.

trained in dance technique. After St. Denis and Shawn separated, each went their own way. St. Denis became interested in religious dance, while Shawn organized a group of young male dancers, which he again took on tour.[11] In this later period, Shawn also wrote a number of books on dance and was the founder-director of Jacob's Pillow School for Dance in Lee, Massachusetts — a school that still has an annual summer dance workshop.[12]

Martha Graham was born in 1898 in Pennsylvania, although she was raised in California. She was a student of Denishawn and a dancer in that company. In 1923, she left the security of this group to find her own way in the modern dance world; one of her first jobs was teaching modern dance for the Eastman School of Music in Rochester.[13] Soon, she began presenting her own concerts, and she became known for her stark, angular movement style. Throughout her lifetime, Martha Graham has created well over 100 dances and is considered one of the most prolific choreographers on the modern dance scene.

A Graham choreography usually tells a story, although specific subject matter has varied widely from episodes of American frontier life to stories from English literature; Greek myths have also been favorite motifs for many of Graham's works.[14] Her costumes and sets were unique and were frequently designed by leading artists of the day, such as sculptor Isamu Noguchi. The music for Graham's choreographies was also done especially for her dances by many leading modern composers so that the total effect was one of a fusing of the various arts of dance, costuming, sets, and music to produce a dynamic whole that often projected intense symbolism, mystifying illusions, or deep psychological overtones.[15] Graham herself danced the title roles in her works for many years until she finally retired from performing in 1969.

Through her teaching, Martha Graham developed a distinctive technical training system that was innovative in its time. This system was based on the idea of contracting or curving in the center of the body, then releasing these contractions; using the floor as part of gesture through the many falls that she invented; and creating turns having a changing axis.[16] Today, the Graham Company is still one of the most prominent of the modern dance troupes in this country.

Two other modern dance pioneers, Doris Humphrey and Charles Weidman, received their early training and performance experience with the Denishawn group. Humphrey and Weidman left Denishawn in 1928 to go to New York City, where they opened their own dance studio and began their own small performing group. In terms of choreographic style, Humphrey and Weidman differed a great deal. Humphrey excelled in creating large group compositions. Often her concern was mainly pure movement design, but usually her dances showed sympathy for human

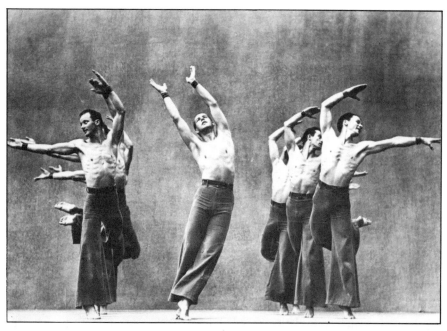

Ted Shawn (center) photographed with his men's dance group performing **Kinetic Molpai** *in 1936. Photo by Shapiro, courtesy of the Dance Collection, The New York Public Library at Lincoln Center*

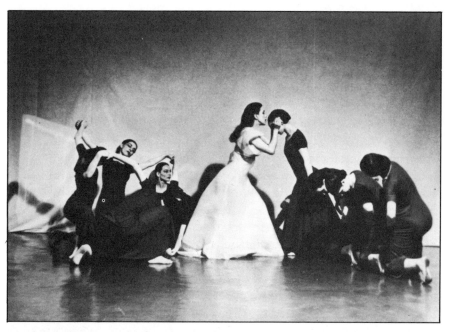

Martha Graham (center) in **Primitive Mysteries**, *circa 1931. Courtesy of the Dance Collection, The New York Public Library at Lincoln Center.*

suffering and a hope for bettering these conditions.[17] Some of Humphrey's works are considered classics of modern dance choreography today. Weidman, on the other hand, had a talent for comic and satiric dances.[18]

Doris Humphrey had considerable talents as a teacher as well. She wrote a book called *The Art of Making Dances*, in which she explained the basis of her choreographic methods. The theory of dance movement that she evolved was based on the process of falling and recovering from falling — a spatial movement pathway that Humphrey discovered between balanced and unbalanced states.[19]

A German form of modern dance had been developing since Duncan had danced in that country in the early 1900s. A name synonymous with the evolution of German modern dance was that of Mary Wigman.

Wigman was born in 1886. Her early training was with Jacques Dalcroze, a Swiss composer and music teacher who devised a system of studying music that involved developing a physical sense of rhythm; and with Rudolf Von Laban, who developed a theoretical system of analyzing human movement. By 1926, she had set up her own school and later started a performing group.

Wigman personified the German nature in her art. Her choreographies, or "dance cycles," were often concerned with basic human emotions. Frequently, Wigman's works appeared mystical or grotesque, and many thought of her as having a preoccupation with dancing about death.[20] The style of these dances was primitive, using rudimentary movements such as crawling, crouching, and creeping.[21] Space was very important and was something to be resisted, while costuming and accompaniment were extremely simple; Wigman often danced without music or to a single woodwind or percussion instrument.[22] Her technical training system used very basic actions and included some improvisation.[23]

Hanya Holm was an early Wigman dancer and student. In 1931, she brought the German style of modern dance to the United States. Holm adapted quickly to American life and settled here permanently. During her lifetime, she has made extensive contributions to the American modern dance, particularly through her teaching and choreography.[24] Many well-known dancers and dance educators have been her students at one time. Holm has also done the choreography for Broadway musicals, including *Kiss Me Kate* and *My Fair Lady*, and each summer she is the guiding force behind a summer dance institute held at Colorado College in Colorado Springs. Together with Graham, Humphrey, Weidman, and composer Louis Horst, Holm contributed to the Bennington School of Dance, which hosted some of the first summer dance festivals from 1934

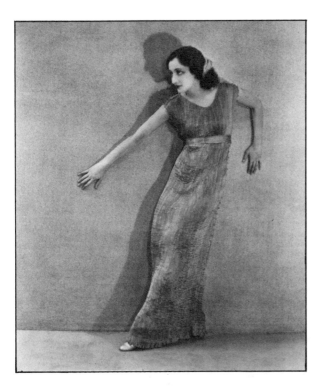

Doris Humphrey, circa
1929. A study by Soichi
Sunami courtesy of the
Dance Collection, The
New York Public Library
at Lincoln Center.

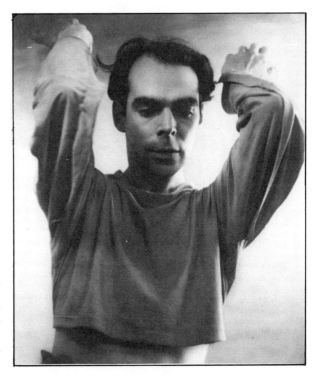

Charles Weidman in
Danse Profane.
Photograph by Hewett
courtesy of the Dance
Collection, The New York
Public Library at Lincoln
center.

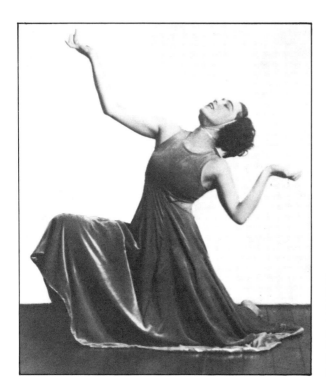

Mary Wigman in
**Schwingende
Landschoft,** 1929.
Uncredited German photo
courtesy of the Dance
Collection, The New York
Public Library at Lincoln
Center.

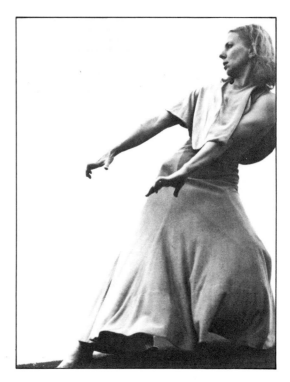

Hanya Holm performing
Trends, 1937. Courtesy
of the Dance Collection,
The New York Public
Library at Lincoln Center.

to 1942. This festival, like many of those that now exist, gave dance an educational focus so that many young people became acquainted with the modern dance in a college setting.[25]

Each of the pioneering individuals of modern dance was unique, developing his/her own choreographic mode of expression and technical training system. They all felt it was their right as modern dancers to pursue their own movement style and expressive direction.

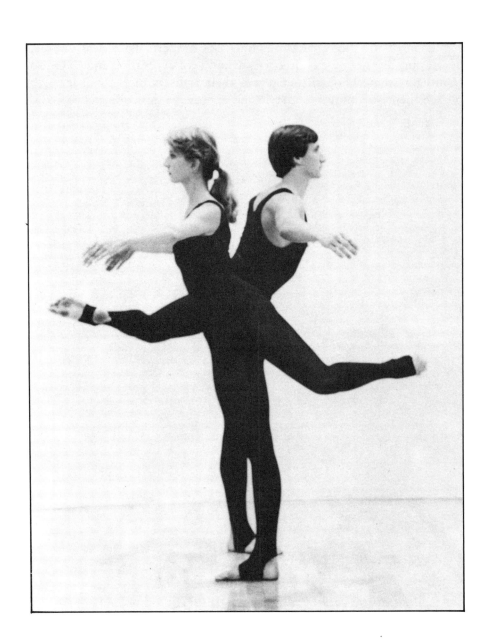

CHAPTER 2

Knowing Your Body

A knowledge of the structure and function of the body can improve dance ability by making you aware of movement potential or restrictions at different places in the body.

The Skeleton

The skeletal framework (Figures 2-1 through 2-3) is formed by many bones that are joined together in a variety of ways. Some of these joints, such as those between the bones of the skull or between the bones of the pelvis, are fused or nearly fused together and are not important in dance movement.

The joints that are important to the dance student are known as synovial joints (Figure 2-4). They are surrounded by fibrous tissue and are filled with a lubricating fluid called synovial fluid.[1] There are four types of synovial joints, each providing a difference in movement potential depending on its location in the skeletal framework and its specific shape. These four types of joints are named according to the number of directions in which movement is possible. They are known as: (1) nonaxial or gliding joints; (2) uniaxial joints; (3) biaxial joints; and (4) triaxial joints. In a nonaxial joint, the separate bones simply glide or slide over each other. An example of a nonaxial joint would be between the individual bones that comprise parts of the foot[2] (Figure 2-5). Uniaxial joints provide for motion in only one direction. The elbow and knee are uniaxial or hinge joints (Figure 2-6).[3] The wrist has two-directional movement and is consequently biaxial[4] (Figure 2-7). Finally, joints providing for potential movement in three directions are called ball-and-socket or triaxial joints. They are similar in shape to a ball on the end of one bone, which fits into a cup-shaped socket in the adjacent bone. Triaxial joints provide for the greatest range of movement in the human body and are found at the shoulder and hip (Figure 2-8).[5]

Synovial joints are reinforced by ligaments that attach one bone to another, and by muscles and their tendon attachments to the bones.[6] If a joint is forced beyond normal range, injury usually occurs in the form of

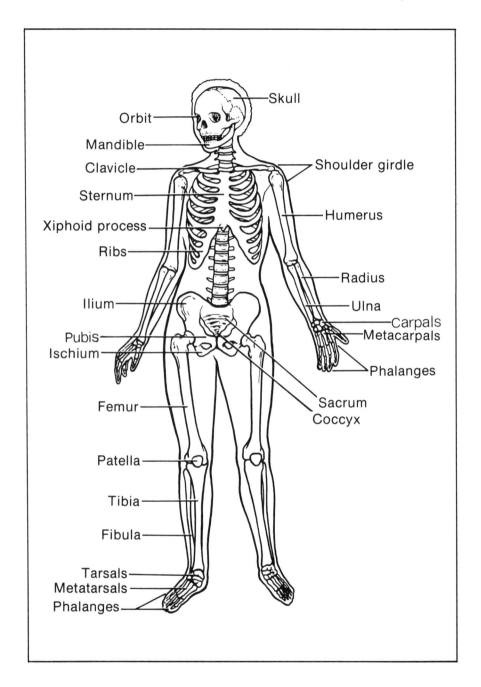

Figure 2-1
Major bones of skeleton involved in alignment and weight bearing. Front view.

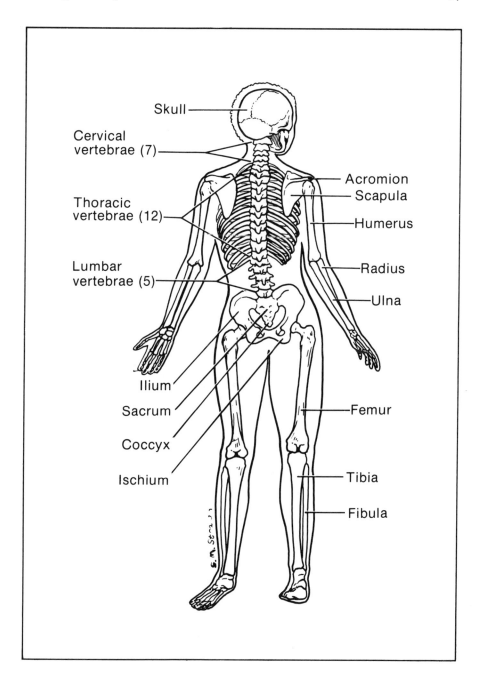

Figure 2-2
Major bones of the skeleton involved in alignment and weight bearing. Back view.

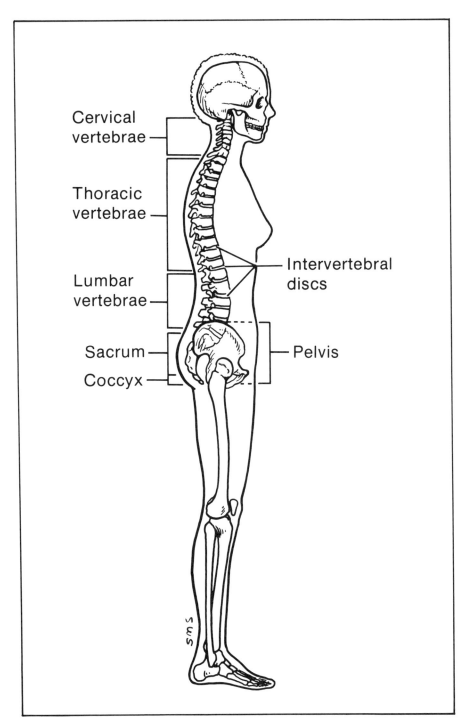

Figure 2-3
Major bones of skeleton involved in alignment and weight bearing. Side view.

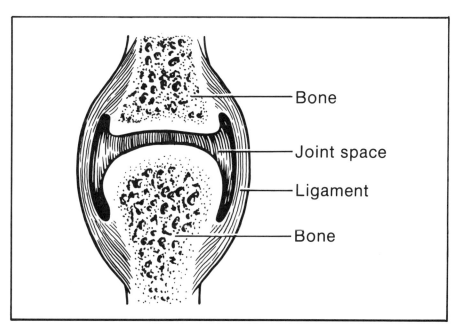

Figure 2-4
Diagram of a synovial joint.

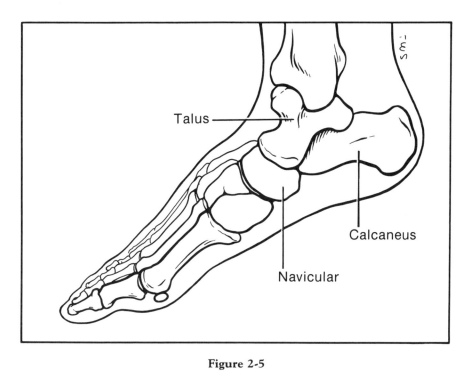

Figure 2-5
The articulations between the talus, calcaneus and navicular are examples of nonaxial joints.

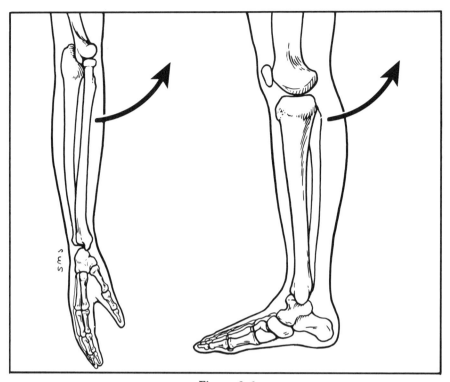

Figure 2-6
Uniaxial or hinge joints in the knee and elbow.

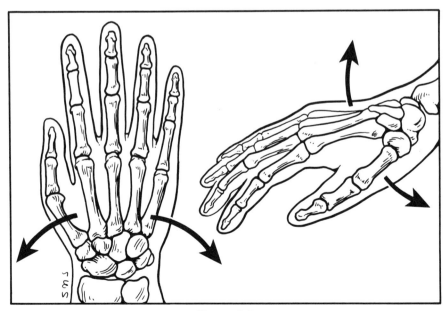

Figure 2-7
The wrist is a biaxial joint.

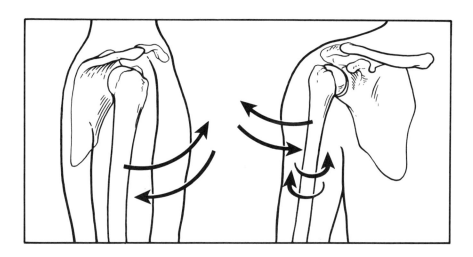

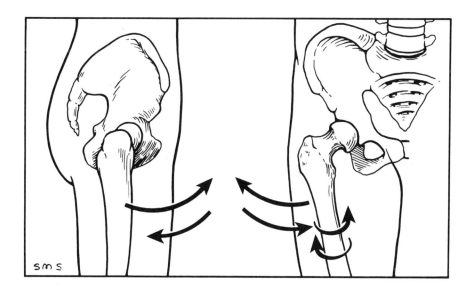

Figure 2-8
Triaxial or ball and socket joints of the shoulder and the hip.

strained or torn muscles, pulled tendons, overly stretched or torn ligaments, or even dislocated joints. It takes time for injuries to heal, and those that are not cared for properly, or those that become chronic, can cause a buildup of scar tissue during the healing process and may permanently impair the range of movement in an area.[7] Caution and proper warm-up are advised to help avoid such injuries.

Muscles and Movement

The tendon attachment of a muscle spans or crosses a joint at many locations within the body, and when the fibers that make up a muscle shorten or contract, movement is produced (Figure 2-9). The nature and direction of the resulting movement are determined by the placement of the muscle in relation to each joint.[8] In dance, we are concerned with groups of muscles and their resulting actions, rather than with individual muscles. These muscles and their resulting movements are best understood when seen as paired groups located on opposite sides of body segments. In the upper arm, there are the biceps at the front of the arm and the triceps at the back; the various sets of abdominal muscles are located at the front of the body, with the muscles of the back on the opposite side of the torso. In the leg segments, there are the hamstrings at the back of the thigh which are paired with the quadriceps group at the front, and the gastrocnemius and soleus at the back of the lower leg opposite the tibialis anterior and other muscles at the front of the lower leg (Figures 2-10 through 2-11).

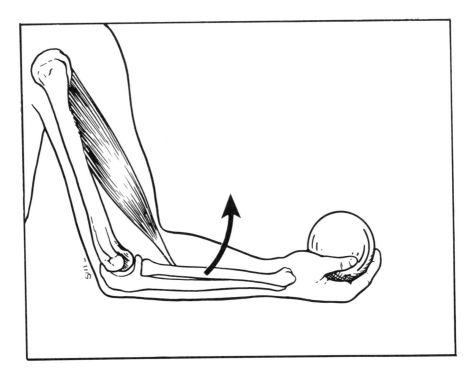

Figure 2-9
Diagram of a muscle and its tendon attachment crossing joint.

In dance, each action has many different names, but the simplest method of identifying movements is to use the anatomically correct names. These names are as follows:

1. Flexion is to narrow the angle at a joint.[9] We can flex at the shoulder, elbow, hip, and knee (Figures 2-12 through 2-13). To flex the ankle is known as dorsiflexion — usually simply called flexion in dance class (Figure 2-14). Flexion is also possible in the center of the body in the spine[10] (Figures 2-15 through 2-16).

2. Extension means to straighten at a joint and is a return from flexion; and to go beyond normal extension is to hyperextend in that area[11] (Figure 2-17). Hyperextension is a common problem in dance, particularly in the knees and lower back (Figures 2-18 through 2-19). Extending the ankle is actually called plantar flexion (Figure 2-20).

3. To abduct at a joint is to move the segment away from the midline of the body.[12] Figure 2-21 is an example of abduction at the shoulder and the hip.

4. A return of a segment toward the middle of the body is known as adduction[13] (Figure 2-22). The terms abduction and adduction are not used as frequently in dance as are the words flexion and extension.

5. Rotation is a twisting movement around a line or long axis that runs through the center of the bony segment being twisted.[14] Rotation is possible in triaxial joints such as the shoulder and hip and also occurs between the separate bones or vertebrae of the spine (Figures 2-23 through 2-27). When a twisting or rotation occurs in the bones of the foot, it is known as eversion or inversion[15] (Figures 2-28 through 2-29). In dance, we simply talk about rolling inward, or to the outer border of the foot, rather than using the words eversion or inversion.

Dance movement typically occurs in longer sequences than the individual actions described in the preceding section. In addition, one movement flows or feeds into the next, often making analysis and learning difficult for the beginner. When watching a class demonstration, the beginning dancer is often bewildered by the array of motions performed by the instructor. Confusion can be reduced by knowing the movement potential of the different joints and by being able to see which type of movement, such as flexion, extension, or rotation, is being performed.

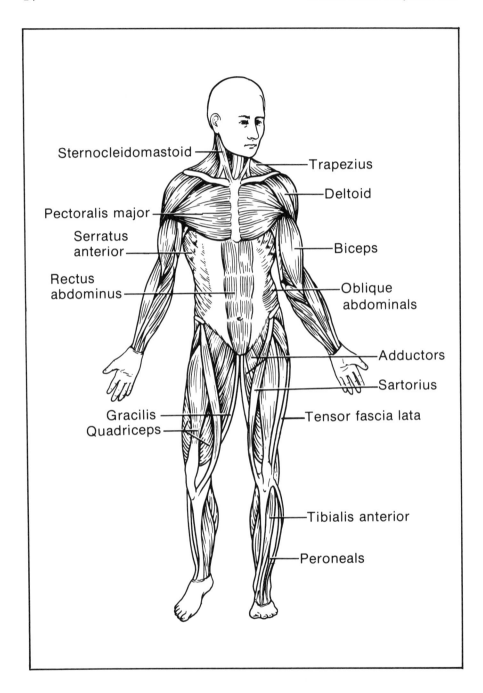

Figure 2-10
Important muscles and muscle groups involved in dancing. Front view.

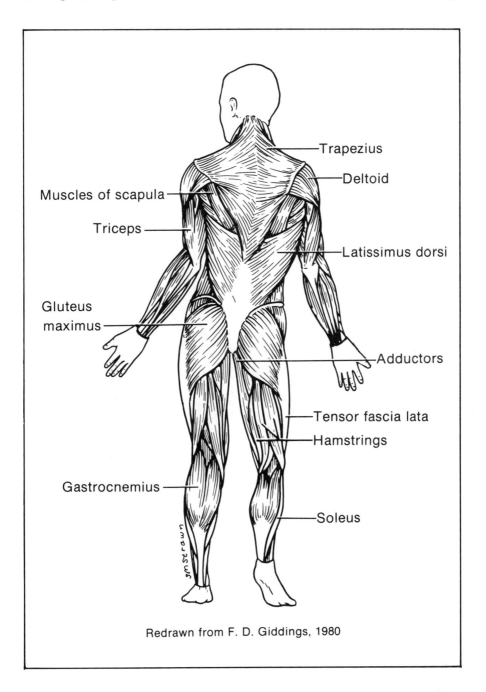

Figure 2-11
Important muscles and muscle groups involved in dancing. Back view.

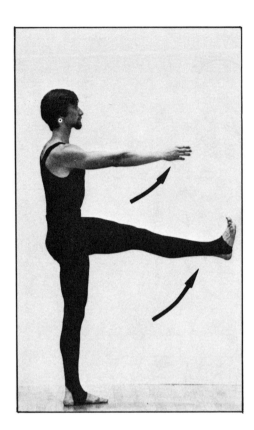

Figure 2-12
Shoulder and hip flexion.

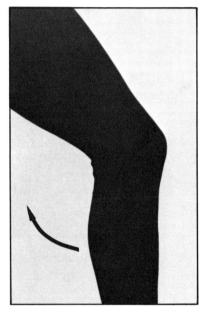

Figure 2-13
Knee flexion.

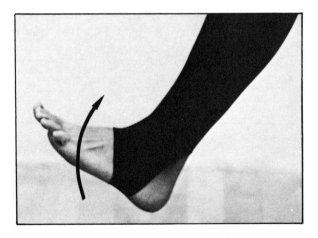

Figure 2-14
Dorsiflexion.

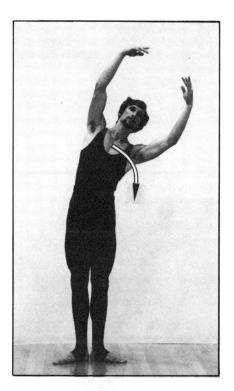

Figure 2-15
Lateral flexion of spine.

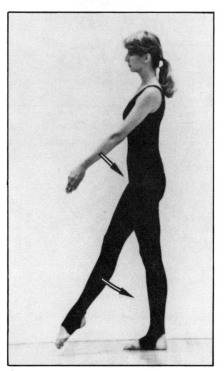

Figure 2-16
Forward flexion of spine.

Figure 2-17
Arrows indicate movement into extension at shoulder and hip.

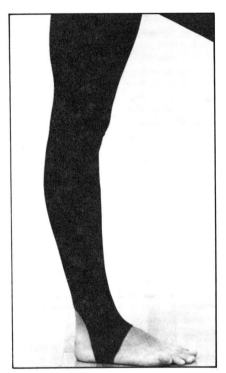

Figure 2-18
Hyperextended knee with knee cap pressed back beyond normal straight or extended position.

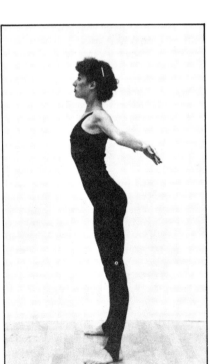

Figure 2-20
Ankle in plantor flexion or extended position.

Figure 2-19
Overarched or hyperextended spine.

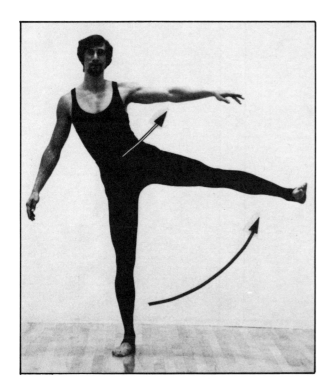

Figure 2-21
*Abduction at shoulder
and hip.*

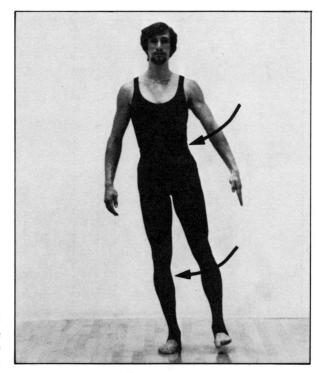

Figure 2-22
*To move toward the
midline of the body is to
adduct.*

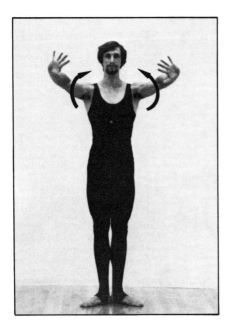

Figure 2-23
Inward rotation at the shoulder.

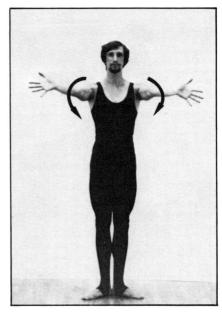

Figure 2-24
Outward rotation at the shoulder.

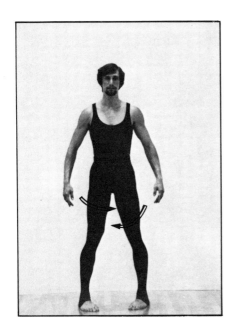

Figure 2-25
Inward rotation in both hips.

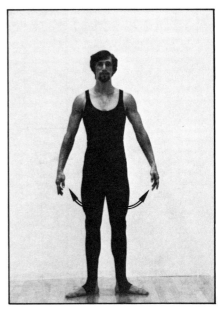

Figure 2-26
Outward rotation in both hips.

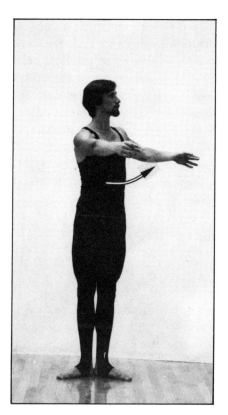

Figure 2-27
Rotation or twisting in the spine.

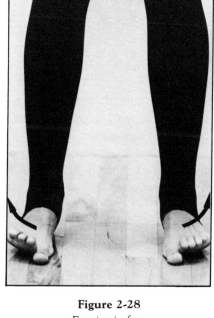

Figure 2-28
Eversion in foot.

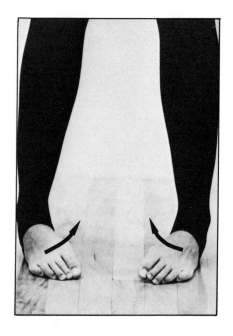

Figure 2-29
Inversion in foot.

Figures 2-30, a-g show a typical modern dance movement sequence that combines many of the individual actions already described. You can see in the first three photos that the dancer is flexing in the hips and knees of both legs, then flexing and curving in the center of the body while moving both arms forward to a flexed position at the shoulders. In the next picture, the forward movement of the body is accompanied by an extension of the knee and ankle of the free leg. These actions are followed by extension of the knee and hip of the supporting leg; falling forward into a lunge position; and cushioning that landing by again flexing in the hip, knee, and ankle of the supporting leg. Finally, the arms open into an abducted position to the side.

Limitations

The potential of the human body for movement is limited by a variety of factors. Some of these limitations, such as the type of joint structure, the location of muscles and their tendons and ligaments, and the attachments of these structures to bones, have already been discussed. In addition, human movement potential is limited by the shape of your entire body.

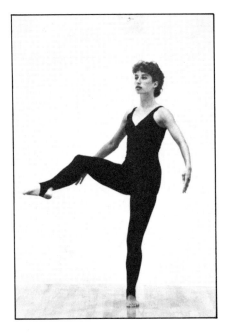

Figure 2-30a
The series of photos, a-g, shows a typical modern dance movement sequence. In the picture at left the dancer is flexing the hips and knees of both legs.

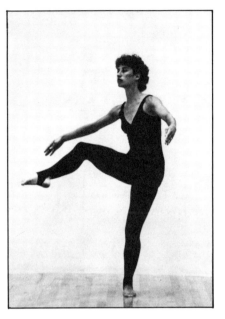

Figure 2-30b

The center of the body curves as the spine flexes forward.

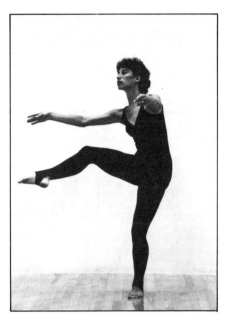

Figure 2-30c

Both arms are flexed forward from the shoulders.

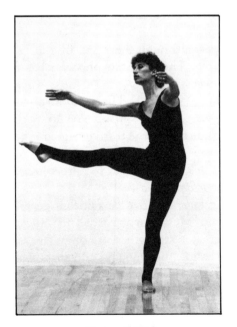

Figure 2-30d

The knee and ankle of the nonweighted leg are extended.

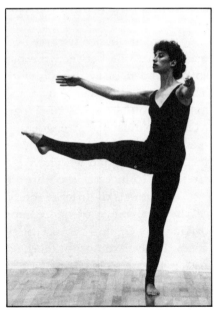

Figure 2-30e

Extension of the knee and hip of the supporting leg follow.

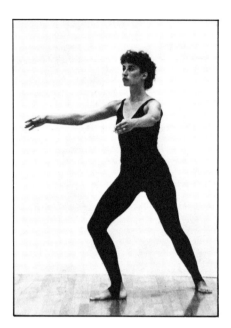

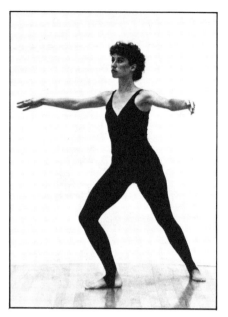

Figure 2-30f

The dancer lunges forward flexing the hip, knee, and ankle of forward leg in order to cushion the landing.

Figure 2-30g

The arms are opened to the side into an abducted position.

There are basically three body types, although there are, of course, many variations between the basic three. The endomorph, who has a soft, rounded body, usually with an excess of fatty tissue, must work harder to acquire endurance and control weight.[16] The ectomorph is long, lean, and loosely strung together; people in this group have to work to develop muscular strength and endurance.[17] In the third group are the mesomorphs, who are husky and large boned, usually of short or medium height, and who have bulky, thick muscles that require a lot of stretching to increase mobility[18] (Figures 2-31, a-c).

Individuals of differing body types have distinct capacities in terms of the total range of dance movement. Mesomorphs excel in quick, darting movements because of their greater strength and compactness. The willowy ectomorph, on the other hand, finds languid and sustained patterns more to his/her liking.

Many individual differences outside of the three basic body types also exist in terms of the shape of parts of the body. Some people, for example, have swayed or curved backs. In a dance class, such students will be able to correct their swayback to some extent but will never match the straight alignment of the dancer who has a relatively flat spine. The short-legged dancer will find quick movements easy because he/she is stable and close to the floor, but that individual will not be able to perform extended leg circles to equal those of long-legged persons. Likewise, people with long backs can usually perform a modern dance contraction or curving in the center of the body more easily than individuals with a short torso, since they simply have more space in which to move the spine.

Examples of individual structural differences are numerous. You need only view the average beginning modern dance class to see many examples of variation in body type. The important point for you is that it is necessary to work within the limitations of your own body. Emphasis should be placed on personal capabilities and strengths, rather than dwelling on limitations, in order to find your full movement potential.

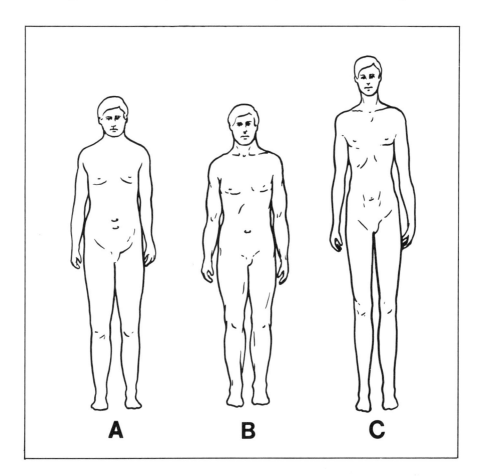

Figure 2-31

*Three types of physique as classified by Sheldon. **A**, Endomorph. **B**, Mesomorph. **C**, Ectomorph.*

Taking Care of Your Body

Good nutrition is extremely important no matter what activities you are involved in during your daily life. If you expect to dance or participate in other physical exercise activities, it is even more important to have a balanced diet.

Food intake should include substances from the four basic food groups each day. These include milk or milk products; meats, fish, and poultry; cereals or grains; and fruits and vegetables. It is recommended that you eat at least two daily servings of milk products and two servings per day of foods from the meat group. Dried beans, peas, nuts, seeds, and eggs can be substituted for meat, fish, or poultry, since these foods contain protein, too. The cereal and grain group provides carbohydrates and should include four daily servings. You also need four servings of fruits and vegetables each day. Plenty of liquids, particularly water, are important to supplement fluid loss in perspiration and to help eliminate waste products from your system. You should drink four to six glasses of water per day.[19] Some dancers and athletes also prefer to take vitamin supplements to help their endurance and energy level. These can be beneficial but should not be taken in excessive amounts. If you decide to take vitamins, select a brand that contains all of the important minerals. When in doubt about vitamins, ask your doctor.

It is important for those wishing to dance to be relatively slim. Excess weight is unattractive in dance clothing and makes it difficult for the dancer to move with ease and efficiency. Weight can be lost by either increasing energy expenditure through exercise or by decreasing caloric intake. The most effective procedure is to reduce food intake and to increase exercise at the same time in order to burn more calories and firm up the body. The most important idea in reducing weight, however, is that the diet still contain sufficient intake of all essential nutrients. You can cut down on helpings at each meal but continue to eat enough servings per day from each food group. Foods such as jellies, cakes, pies, and salad dressings and beverages such as alcohol are high in calories and low in nutritional value. Give yourself a significant time in which to lose weight, since losing a couple of pounds per week is enough. It is recommended that a working dancer have at least 2,000 calories each day in the diet.[20] A good way to calculate your appropriate caloric intake is to multiply your current weight by 12 if you are sedentary; by 15 if you are active and work out on your own or walk a lot; and by 20 if you perform manual labor.[21] To lose weight, you must eat less calories than this number, probably decreasing your intake by about 500 to 1,000 calories per day to lose one to two pounds per week. Avoid fad diets and weight loss pills.

The body needs adequate rest as well as good food in order to function efficiently. Most people require seven to eight hours of sleep each night. Sound nutrition and sufficient rest will reduce the risk of injury and will enable the body to rebuild and repair itself.

Common Injuries

Injuries are usually accompanied by immediate pain and a degree of bleeding in the tissues. Swelling may also occur, but the amount of swelling is not always indicative of the severity of the injury. Pain is the body's way of telling you to stop activity. You should see a doctor concerning the severity of an injury.

Cramps frequently occur when a muscle becomes overly fatigued. A cramp is due to a muscle contracting maximally and remaining in contraction. Pressure should be applied to a cramped muscle by grasping it firmly, rather than massaging it, until cramping subsides, followed by gradual stretching.[22] A lack of salt or fluids in the diet can also cause muscle cramps. A more serious cramping is a spasm of the muscle, lasting for a longer time. Massage, particularly in the back, can help relieve spasms.

A **strain** is a common dance injury that results from excessive stretching of a muscle, causing tearing of muscle fibers. Strains can range from a mild pull involving tearing of only a small number of muscle fibers to a severe pull in which there is a complete rupture of the muscle or of the tendon of that muscle from the adjoining bone.[23] Strains should be treated by applying cold compresses for the first twenty-four to forty-eight hours and by elevating the injured part.[24] Application of cold is followed by heat and rest. A severe pull or strain usually requires surgical repair. Do not try to work out a strain, since this can lead to the formation of scar tissue.

Shin splints are felt as a dull ache in the middle and sometimes at the outside of the lower leg. Generally, they are caused by landing with the heels off the floor and the knees straight, and from dancing on cement floors. A suspended wood floor is recommended for dancing to prevent shin splints. Stretching the front and back of the lower leg before and after activity can be helpful as well.[25] Applying heat is also useful.

Sprains are caused by a joint suddently going beyond its normal range of movement. Characteristically, sprains are a sudden twisting injury accompanied by swelling and immobility in the affected area. A first-degree sprain involves only minor tearing of the ligaments surrounding a joint, while a third-degree sprain is a complete tearing of the supporting ligaments.[26] Sprains require the immediate application of cold, compression, and elevation; any further treatment should be recommended by a physician. Sprains that typically occur in dance are those of the toes, ankles, knees, hips, lower back, and sometimes of the wrists.[27]

It is common for beginning dancers to develop **bruises** when landing incorrectly from jumps or from performing falls improperly. A bruise can result from a direct blow to any part of the body, producing bleeding into the tissue. Discoloration and pain result. A bone bruise to the bottom of the foot can be painful if continued attempts are made to land on the injured area. Apply cold to the bruised area and, where possible, stretch the area to relieve muscle spasm.[28]

Blisters are caused by pressure and friction, especially when performing turns with bare feet. Fluid accumulates between the layers of the skin in a localized area; unopened blisters should be padded and covered. If you decide to open a blister, wash the area thoroughly and disinfect it. Sterilize a needle in a flame, and puncture the blister by inserting the needle parallel to skin and close to the edge of the blister. Apply gentle pressure to remove fluid. For about a week, put *Vaseline*® on the punctured blister and cover it with padding that will not stick to the skin. Blood blisters should not be opened, because they become infected more easily.[29]

A thickening of the skin, or **callus,** on the sole of the foot comes about as a protection in response to pressure and friction against the floor. Some callusing is realistic and allows the foot to slide across the floor more easily. Excessive calluses, however, can be caused by poor posture or improper weight bearing. Calluses can be reduced by filing them down with an emery board or by softening them with lanolin.[30]

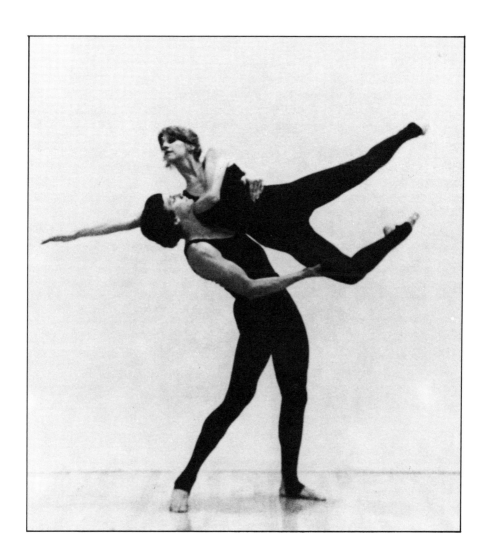

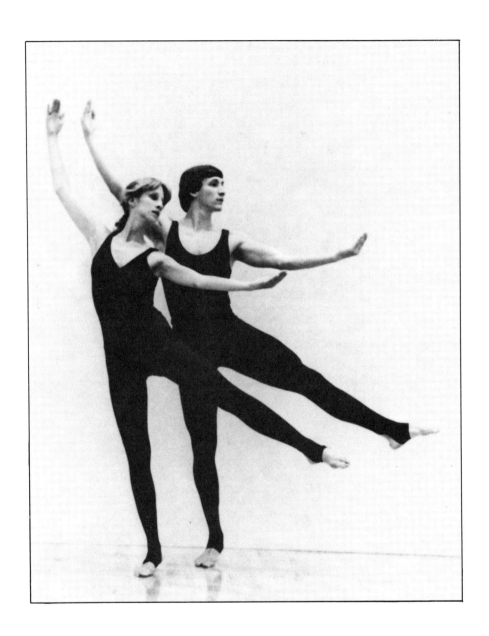

CHAPTER 3

The Dance Class

Goals of a Beginning Modern Dance Class

Alignment

A good understanding of correct body alignment is extremely important for the beginning dancer, since good alignment — whether it is sitting or standing — is the place from which all movement begins. In correct alignment, a straight line can be visualized as going through a series of points when the body is viewed in profile. This line, which is sometimes known as the line of gravity, goes just behind the ear, through the center of the shoulder and hip joints, a little in front of the ankle, and down through the foot[1] (Figure 3-1). You can easily experience correct alignment by lying on your back and visualizing the line of gravity going through all of the points mentioned above.

Good alignment can also be evaluated from the front or back of the body. From either of these viewpoints, the shoulders and hips should appear level in a well-aligned body. The knees should be at the same level from the floor, with the weight placed evenly on both feet. Rolling in on the arches or to the outer border of the foot should be avoided in any dance movement or position where one or two feet are placed flat on the floor. Generally, a triangular weight placement is recommended with three points — the inner border of the ball of the foot, the outer border of the ball of the foot, and the middle of the heel — placed firmly on the floor[2] (Figure 3-2).

When you begin to move, total alignment will naturally tilt in the direction of the movement to facilitate the desired momentum. In motion, however, alignment is maintained so that the body still has as unbroken a line as possible (Figures 3-3, a-b). The degree to which the dancer must tilt to increase momentum depends on the speed of the movement being performed so that, for example, a run would require a greater forward tilt than a walk.

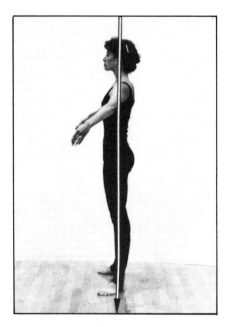

Figure 3-1
The line of gravity in correct alignment.

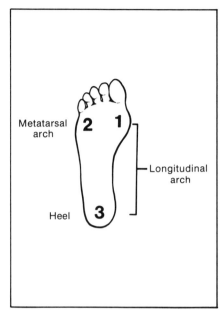

Figure 3-2
Drawing showing correct weight placement when the foot is flat on the floor.

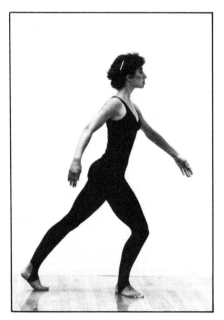

Figure 3-3a
A dance walk in which good alignment is maintained.

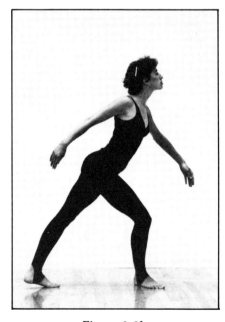

Figure 3-3b
A poor dance walk with a forward head, and the hips too far back.

Gravity

Another necessary aspect of learning to dance is understanding how to move efficiently in relation to gravity. As long as you move on this earth, you will have to contend with the pull of gravity. In correct alignment in dance, you need to lift the center of the body away from gravity. The center of the body is found at the center of gravity, the most dense point in the body, located in the middle of the pelvic area.[3] In women, the center of gravity is generally lower than it is in men because of the shorter stature and wider hips.

In beginning dance classes, emphasis is placed on learning to lift the center so that the weight is not dropped into the legs. This relieves the legs of considerable stress and gives you a look and feeling of lightness. Lifting the center also enables you to move, stop, and change directions easily and with greater agility.

Dance movements are performed much more effectively if done with a lifted center. For example, a grand plié is a dance warmup in which the individual bends the knees slowly until a deep knee bend is achieved (Figure 3-4). Recovery from the grand plié would be much more difficult if the dancer did not have a lifted center, since all the weight would be into the floor and all the momentum would be lost in the legs and feet (Figure 3-5). With the center lifted, momentum is saved for the upward part or recovery portion of the movement, facilitating the ascent.

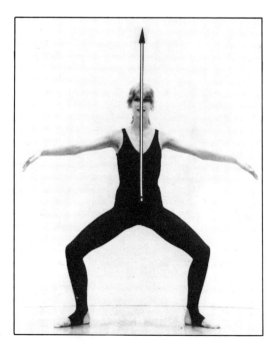

Figure 3-4
A plié with the center lifted.

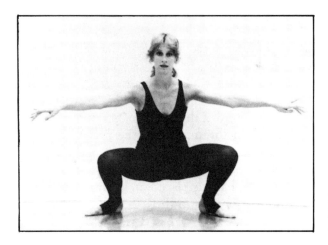

Figure 3-5
Incorrect plié with center dropped toward floor.

A modern dance fall is also done more efficiently with the center lifted. On the downward part of the fall, it is again important to continue to lift the center to keep the body from giving in to gravity too rapidly. If the lift is not maintained throughout the downward part of the movement, injury could occur upon hitting the floor, and recovery on the upward part of the action would again be very difficult (Figures 3-6, a-d).

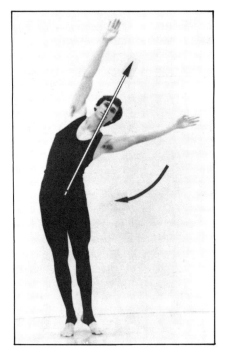

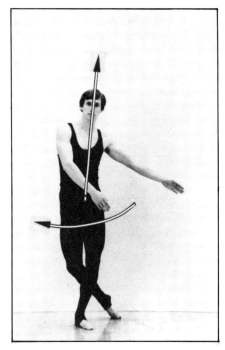

Figure 3-6a
A modern dance fall to the side. Arrows indicate lifted center and direction of movement.

Figure 3-6b

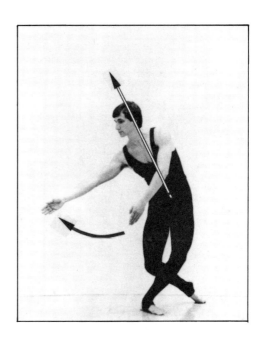

Figure 3-6c

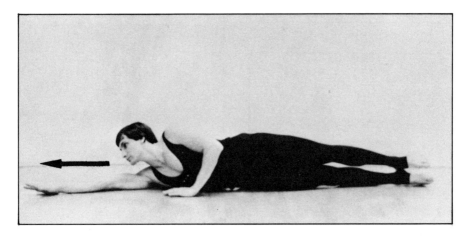

Figure 3-6d

In some dance movements, gravity can be helpful, and energy can be saved if the dancer gives in to gravity while performing the action. The swing is a popular modern dance movement in which gravity can be an aid. In fact, if the dancer does not drop with gravity on the downward portion of the movement, the swing will not be done properly, because there will be too much tension in the downward arc of the swing in an effort to resist the pull of gravity (Figures 3-7, a-c).

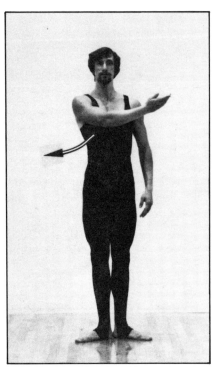

Figure 3-7a

In an arm swing gravity helps initiate the downward part of the arc.

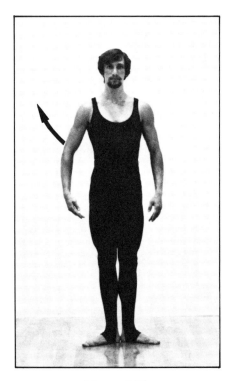

Figure 3-7b

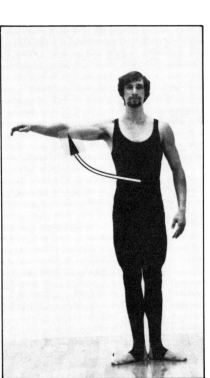

Figure 3-7c

The dancer needs to apply energy to complete the upward part of the swinging action.

Balance

Gaining a better sense of balance is another aspect of dance technique. Balancing has to do with: (1) alignment and stability and (2) with directing energies in the body.

A dancer with a lower center of gravity is much more stable than one with the center of gravity located higher in the body.[4] This makes the grand plié second position extremely secure and a good position in which to stop the body following rapid movement or turning. The wide base of support, also found in the grand plié in second position, adds to the stability, since the narrower the base of support, the less stable the dance position.[5]

Stability in balancing is decreased when there is less of the underneath surface of the foot on which to balance. Thus, balancing on one foot or in a half toe position is much more difficult. To increase your ability to balance in these positions, keep the center of gravity above the supporting base.[6] This is also important while performing various leg gestures when standing on one foot (Figures 3-8, a-b).

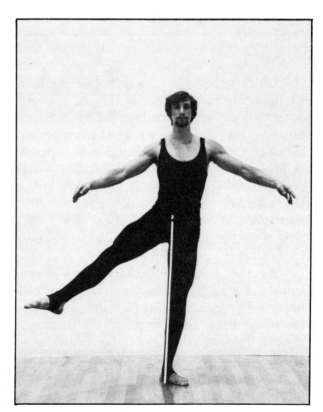

Figure 3-8a
A balance on one leg with center above base.

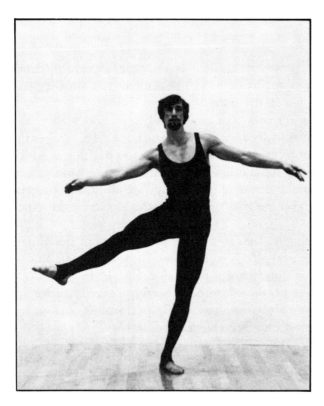

Figure 3-8b
*Incorrect balance with
center shifted to the side of
base.*

Directing body energies appropriately also aids balancing. Generally, we think of these energies as flowing outward from the center of the body. Whenever one part of the body moves away from center, an opposing part has to be stretched in an opposite direction to maintain balance.[7] One example of such directed energies would be to stand in a half toe position on one or two feet. This position is commonly known as a relevé. Balancing in this position becomes easier when you think about sending energy from the center upward. At the same time, you must press down into the floor with a similar amount of energy. Sometimes instructors actually talk about pressing up into a relevé in half toe position (Figure 3-9).

Another example of balancing with directed energies would be the arabesque used in both modern dance and ballet. Here, balance can be improved by concentrating on your energy going up and out through the top of the head, downward into the floor through the supporting leg, backward through the lifted and extended leg, and horizontally out from the center through the arms. Many other examples could be given in which concentration on directed energies can aid balance (Figures 3-10 through 3-11).

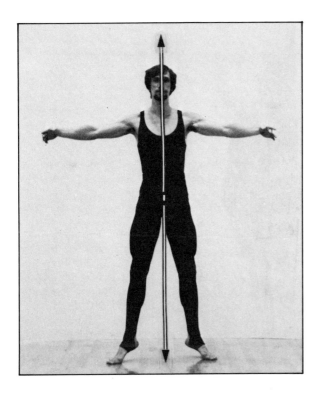

Figure 3-9
Relevé with arrows
indicating how energy
should be directed from
the center.

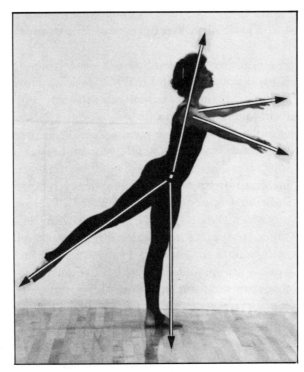

Figure 3-10
Directing the energy
outward from center while
balancing in arabesque.

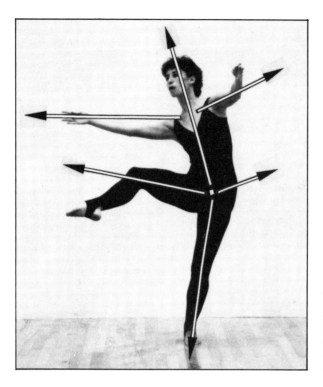

Figure 3-11
In asymmetrical dance positions and movements, energy also radiates outward from the center to help maintain balance.

Flexibility, Strength, and Endurance

Another important part of dance training is understanding how to control your body and make it do what you want it to do at the right time. Such control gradually improves by building good dance skills or technique in the form of increased flexibility, greater strength, and the endurance to continue moving for longer periods of time.

Flexibility means having a greater range of movement in particular joint areas in the body than does the average person. Flexibility is increased by stretching the basic muscles important in dancing so that the individual is not severely restricted in terms of the size of the dance movements to be performed. Stretching is a lengthening action and should take place in the same direction as the placement of muscle fibers being stretched. Figure 3-12 shows a typical stretch for the hamstring muscle group, and Figure 3-13 demonstrates a stretch for the muscles that span the front of the shoulder joint.

Greater strength comes about by making the muscles do more work through a greater number of repetitions of a movement or by holding a position over a longer period of time. Strengthening requires that muscles work by shortening or contracting. In recent years, dancers have

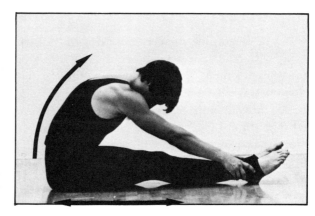

Figure 3-12
A stretch for the hamstring muscles and for the back.

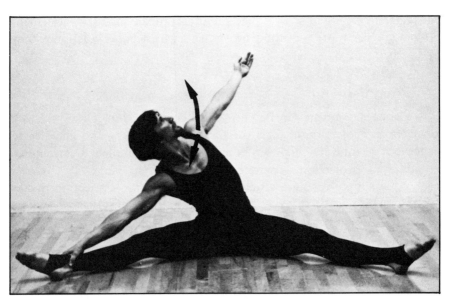

Figure 3-13
Stretching the pectoral muscle at the front of the shoulder.

even begun to lift weights or wear weights on parts of the body as a method of strengthening important muscle groups. It is recommended that strengthening exercises be done through the full range of movement at a joint with a minimum of repetitions and with added resistance.[8]

Increased endurance comes about through greater efficiency of the cardiovascular, respiratory, and muscular systems. Increased endurance, the main thrust in aerobic conditioning or aerobic dancing, is brought about by continuing fast and rapid exercise over increasingly longer periods. All three areas — increased flexibility, strength, and endurance — should be part of a sound modern dance technique class.

Accuracy

The beginning dancer must not only learn how to move his/her body with control but be able to move with accuracy as well. Accuracy in movement comes about with the ability to reproduce a movement as demonstrated by the instructor. Beginning dancers usually need to learn to see movement in terms of body placement and dynamics. The dancer who continues to change the basic feeling and framework of movement from that demonstrated will not be the one later selected for learning a new choreography. What choreographer wants his/her creative work altered by a dancer? Gradually, you should work to gain an overall sense of your body, which will enable you to be aware of the whole and yet sensitive to the positioning of the parts at the same time. As a beginning dancer, you need to develop sensitivity to kinesthetic sensations of muscular tension and spacial placement accompanying each movement so that you can reproduce these movements with accuracy each time they are performed.[9]

Projection

Dance movement can be performed correctly, but it can still lack projection. Projection enables the dancer's movement and energies to reach out beyond his/her own body to touch the audience. An understanding of projection should begin in the first dance class. Good technique simply involves efficient body mechanics. Projection makes technique into dance; it makes dancing come alive. Thus, there should be an inner awareness that is part of each movement and that sparks the observer to respond from within with various tensions in the muscles of his/her own body.[10]

Efficient and correct use of body energies contributes to projection. Isadora Duncan talked about energy emanating from the center of the body. Perhaps she was one of the first dancers to consciously realize that energy flowed into the extremities from the center, and that it was this energy flow that made the body come alive, enabling the dancing to have a sense of projection reaching across space[11] (Figures 3-14, a-b). In many modern dance actions, the energy is also pulled back into the center so that there is a constant coursing inward and flowing outward of energy as the dancer completes one sequence and goes on to another.

Breathing also aids projection and movement aliveness. As a general rule, you should breathe in as you move up and out as you move down; holding the breath will make your dance movements appear rigid and stagnant. Breathing with the movement helps give the dancing an illusion of having a life of its own, so that dancers frequently talk about filling the body or a part of the body with breath.[12]

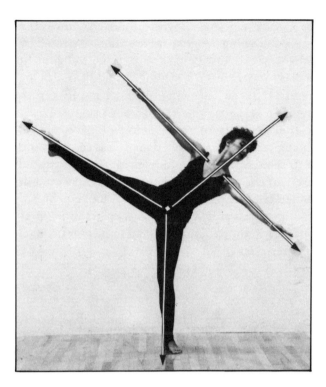

Figure 3-14a
*Modern dance tilt
performed correctly. The
dancer is reaching out
from center to aid
movement projection.*

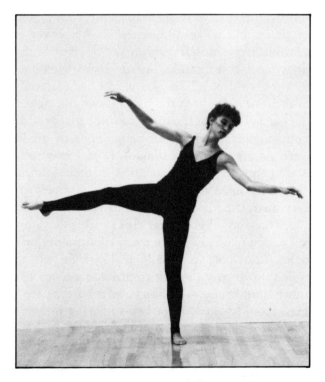

Figure 3-14b
*Incorrect performance of
tilt with no projection.*

Any technique class can become meaningless unless you keep the goals firmly in mind. Simply following dance sequences demonstrated by the teacher is a very mechanical process. Being aware of your alignment or breathing makes the class much more fulfilling. In addition, being conscious of your changing ability in balancing or in accurately reproducing a movement provides a series of checks for your progress.

Awareness of how the elements of movement — space, shape, energy, and time — are being used throughout a dance class can also add interest. You should try to see the size of the movements demonstrated — their sculptural shapes, and the amount of energy and tempo used in each movement. Such understanding of the subtleties of movement can provide added stimulus for progress and help you to see the tremendous variety that you can experience in the sphere of human movement, which makes up the realm of modern dance.

Preparing for Class

It is important to be dressed appropriately for a dance class. Loose clothing gets in the way of movement and can hide the body from view so that your teacher cannot give meaningful corrections.

Women should wear a leotard and tights to class. The leotard color and style are not usually important as long as they hug the body but still allow freedom of movement in all directions. A long-sleeved leotard may be preferable in cold climates. Tights cover the legs, help hold the warmth in the muscles, and make the part of the warm-up done on the floor more comfortable. Stirrup style tights have become very popular for modern dance, because the piece of material that fits under the arch of the foot helps hold the tights down during stretching exercises, while the ball and heel of the foot are still bare for added traction on the floor. Some dancers prefer the original style of modern dance tights, which were simply cut off at the ankle. You may need to wear a bra, and if underpants are worn beneath your dance clothing, they should not be visible. Women should secure their hair before class. Long hair can be very distracting if it is allowed to fall in the face or eyes during class.

Men should also wear close-fitting clothing to class. Stirrup tights are recommended but are made of a heavier material than are women's tights. The tights are usually held up by a belt, with the top of the tights rolled down over the belt to provide a clean visual line. A t-shirt is the most comfortable top. Shirts with buttons are not recommended, and men should wear a dance belt underneath their tights.

Many dance students, both men and women, have begun wearing jazz pants or sweatpants to modern dance classes. The women usually wear these pants over a leotard, and the men tuck their t-shirt into the pants. Such pants are fine but need to be close-fitting, not baggy, so that the body line is in clear view.

Attendance

Attendance and participation are extremely important in dance[1] classes. Reading books about dance technique can be very helpful, but it is essential to practice these movements and experience them in your own body. Doing is learning in dance. Your teacher will probably have his/her own rules concerning attendance.

Class Format

The Warm-Up

Modern dance class usually begins with a warm-up in the center of the dance floor. The purpose of the warm-up is to get the blood circulating and the muscles warmed and stretched. The warm-up is also a time in which the individual psychologically prepares for the more vigorous movement that comes later in the class. In many modern dance classes, the warm-up begins on the floor with the use of large movements reaching from the center of the body. Gradually, the movement is extended out into the legs and arms. Strengthening and stretching exercises — particularly those for the center — are important in the warm-up as well.

The exact design of the warm-up differs from one teacher to another, although each instructor has goals similar to those stated. Your teacher will decide which movements to include in the warm-up in terms of the demands of the remainder of the lesson and the goals of the class. In recent years, some teachers have started lessons with a short quiet time or meditation session so that students can be fully concentrating on their bodies by the time the actual warm-up begins. Some teachers also allow students to do their own mild stretch at the beginning of class to heighten body awareness.

Seated Warm-Up

Many different ways of placing various parts of the body can be found in this part of the warm-up. These positions are illustrated in Figures 3-15, a-m. These positions are not static, but poised in readiness for movement. Frequently, dance sequences also move through these positions during the warm-up.

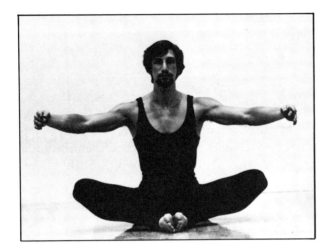

Figure 3-15a
Frog sit.

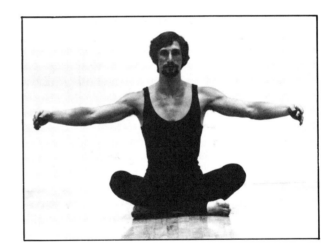

Figure 3-15b
Tailor sit.

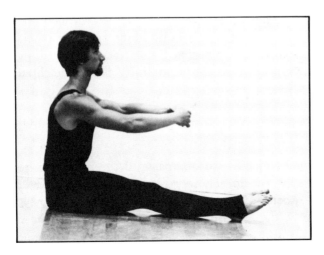

Figure 3-15c
Long sit.

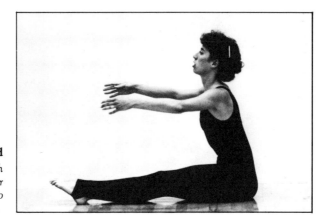

Figure 3-15d
Incorrect long sit with head and shoulders too far forward in relation to hips.

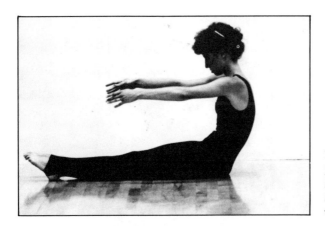

Figure 3-15e
Incorrect long sit with head and shoulders behind hips, and with back rounded.

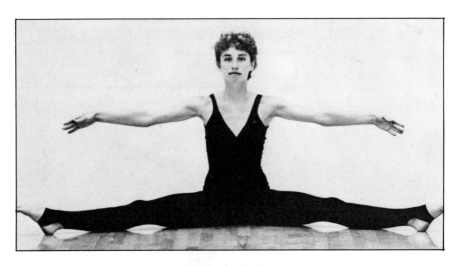

Figure 3-15f
Straddle sit.

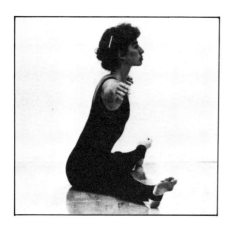

Figure 3-15g
Incorrect straddle rolling into the front of hip joints, and with the head too far forward.

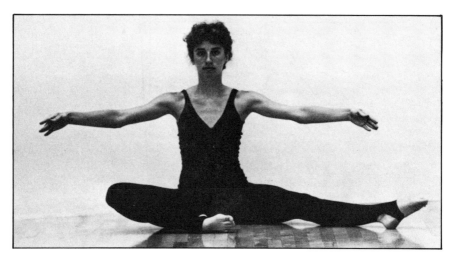

Figure 3-15h
Straddle with one leg flexed at knee.

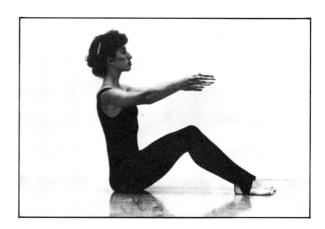

Figure 3-15i
Hook sit.

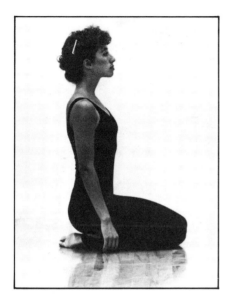

Figure 3-15j
Sitting on the knees.

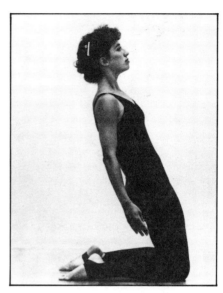

Figure 3-15k
Hinge.

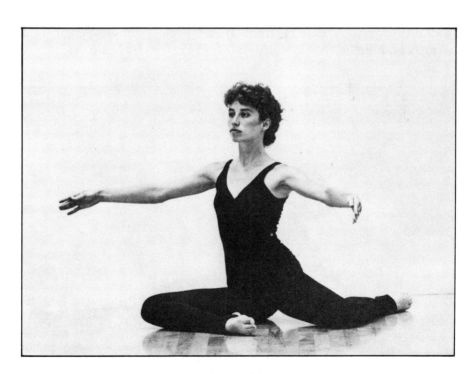

Figure 3-15l
Sitting in fourth position.

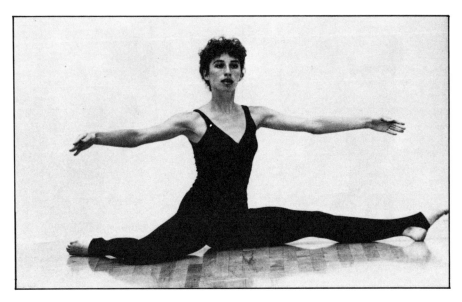

Figure 3-15m
Half split.

Common stretching exercises found in the seated portion of the warm-up are illustrated in Figures 3-16, a-t, while common strengthening sequences done on the floor are shown in Figures 3-17, a-p.

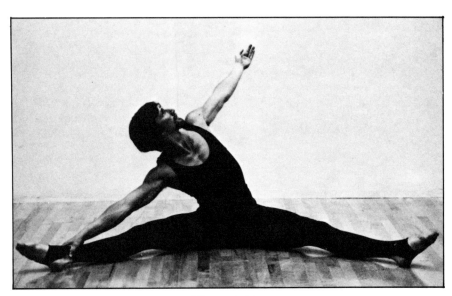

Figure 3-16a
Stretch for pectoral muscle.

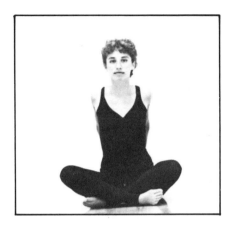

Figure 3-16b
Pectoral muscle stretch.

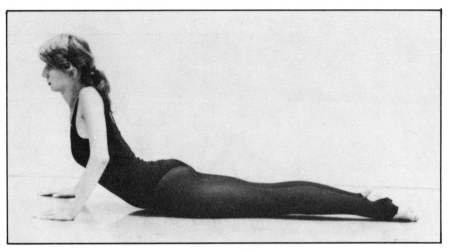

Figure 3-16c
Stretch for the muscles at the front of the body. Care should be taken so that the back does not overarch.

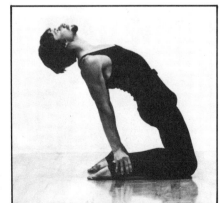

Figure 3-16d
Stretching the abdominal muscles and the quadriceps muscles at the front of the thighs.

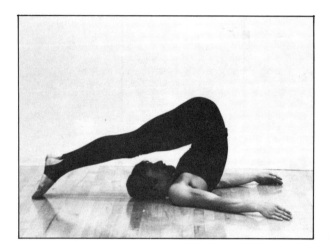

Figure 3-16e
A stretch for the back.

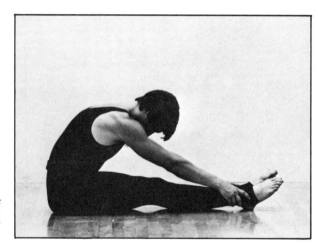

Figure 3-16f
*Stretching the back and
the hamstrings.*

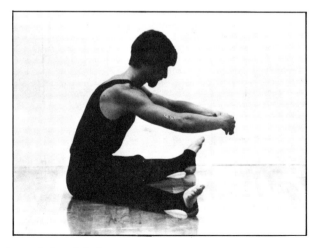

Figure 3-16g
*Stretching the back and
the hamstrings.*

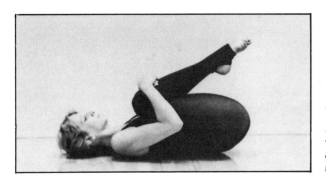

Figure 3-16h
A stretch for the back, recommended for the dancer who is very tight in this area.

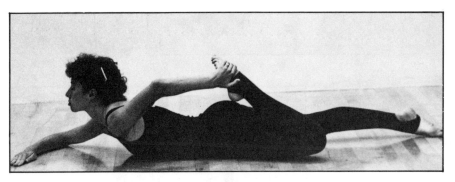

Figure 3-16i
A stretch for the quadriceps.

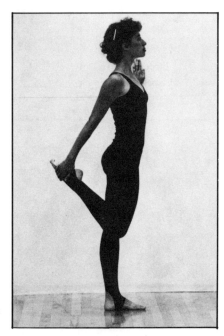

Figure 3-16j
Another stretch for the quadriceps done in a standing position.

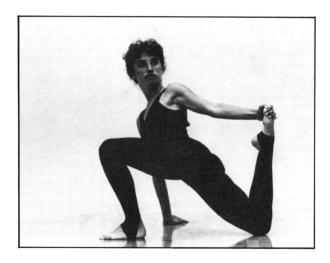

Figure 3-16k
A quadriceps stretch for the more advanced dancer. Also stretches the hamstrings of the opposite leg.

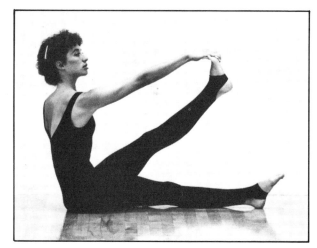

Figure 3-16l
Hamstring stretch.

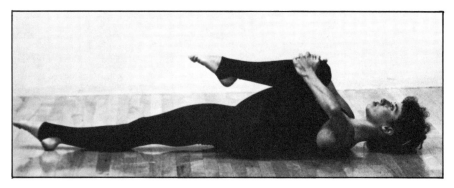

Figure 3-16m
Hamstring stretch with flexed knee.

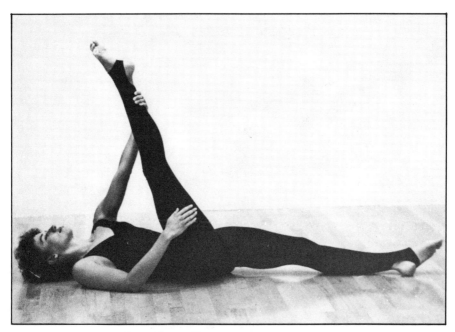

Figure 3-16n
Hamstring stretch with extended knee.

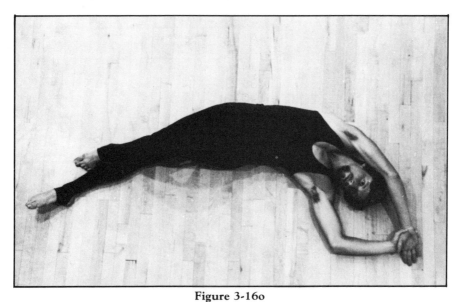

Figure 3-16o
A stretch for the abductor muscles at the outside of the hip joint. (From Fitt, S., Kinesiology for Teachers of Dance class notes, University of Utah, summer 1982).

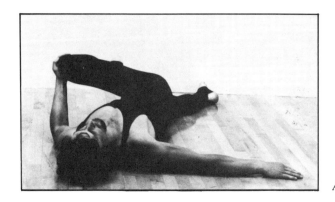

Figure 3-16p
Another abductor stretch.

Figure 3-16q
*The Fitt stretch for the abductors. (From Arnheim, D.: **Dance Injuries, Their Prevention and Care** (St. Louis, The C. V. Mosby Co., 1980), p. 97.*

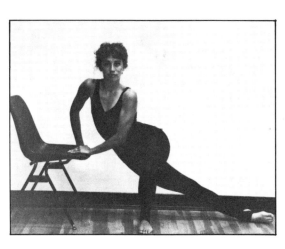

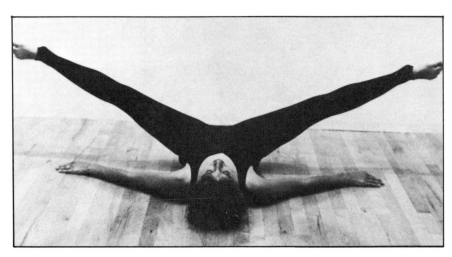

Figure 3-16r
Gravity can be used to help stretch the adductors or inner thigh muscles.

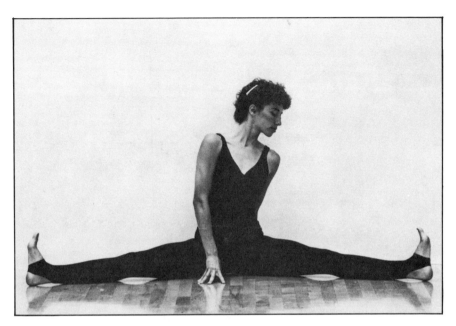

Figure 3-16s

Lifting the hips slightly and pressing forward into a wider straddle sit is another way to stretch adductors.

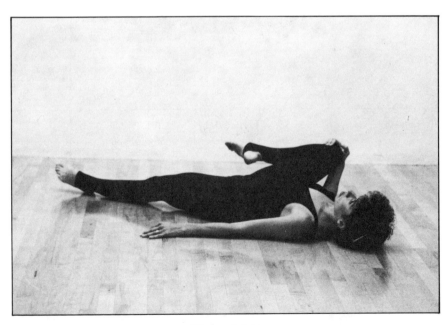

Figure 3-16t

When the leg is pulled on the diagonal to the side, the adductors and the hamstrings are stretched.

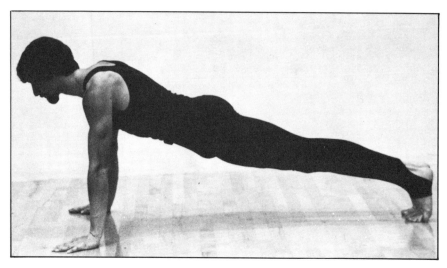

Figure 3-17a

A push-up for strengthening the muscles of the shoulder area.

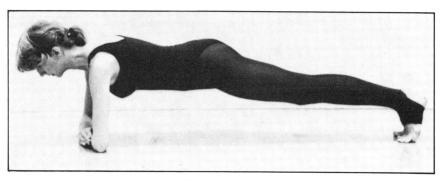

Figure 3-17b

Performing the push-up from the elbows relieves the strain on the wrists.

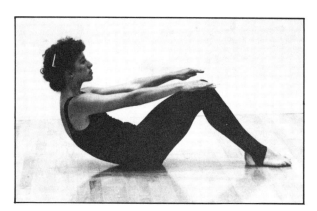

Figure 3-17c

An abdominal curl works the muscles at the front of the body. The knees should be flexed, with the feet flat on floor in parallel position.

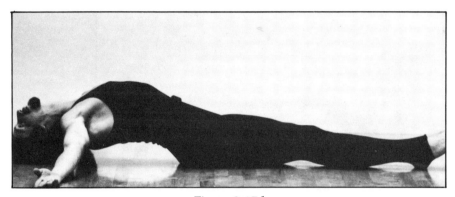

Figure 3-17d

A more advanced abdominal curl is performed by lifting from the sternum first. Care should be taken to avoid overarching the lower back during this action.

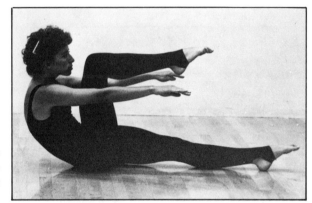

Figure 3-17e

Another variation of the abdominal curl brings the chin to the knee.

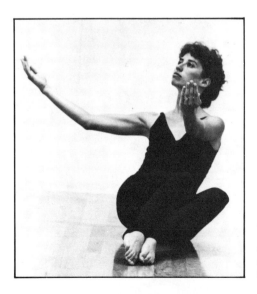

Figure 3-17f

An abdominal curl which twists to the side strengthens the diagonal or oblique abdominal muscles.

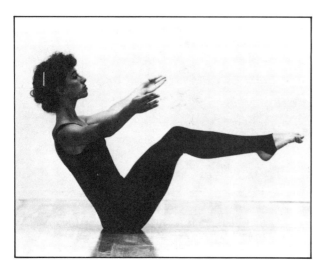

Figure 3-17g
An additional strengthening exercise for the abdominal muscles which is accomplished by lifting the legs and torso off the floor at the same time, with the legs flexing at the knees at the beginning of the movement.

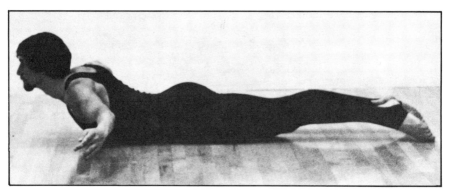

Figure 3-17h
Strengthening the upper back by lifting the upper body off the floor.

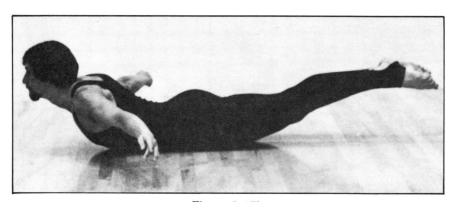

Figure 3-17i
Strengthening the back and the back of the legs.

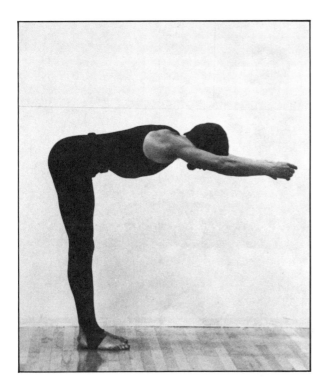

Figure 3-17j
Reaching forward parallel to the floor also strengthens the back.

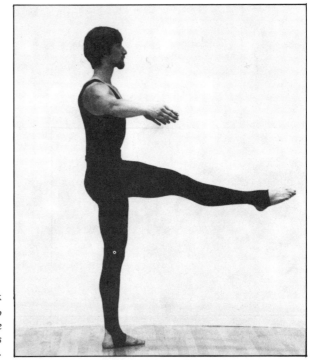

Figure 3-17k
Lifting the leg at the hip directly in front of the body works the quadriceps muscle group.

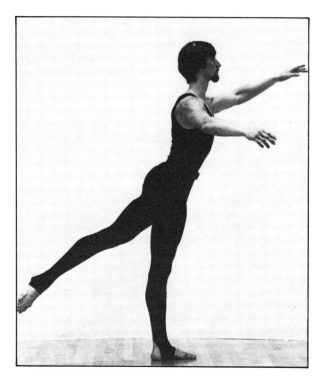

Figure 3-17l
Holding the leg in the above position helps strengthen the hamstring muscles.

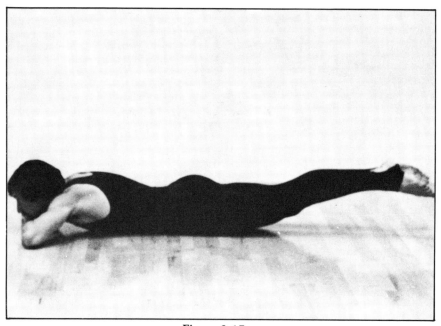

Figure 3-17m
Another strengthening exercise for the hamstrings.

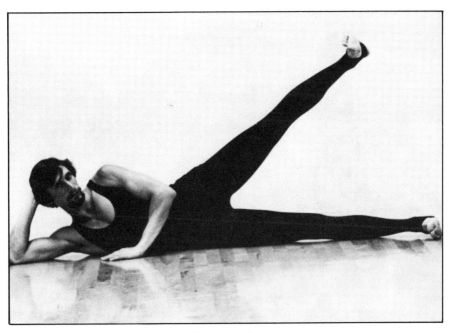

Figure 3-17n

Lifting the leg directly to the side of the body in parallel position helps strengthen the abductors.

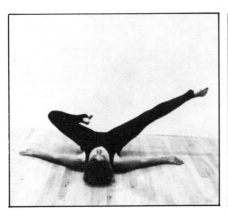 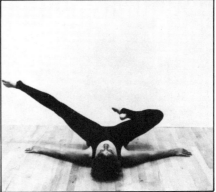

Figure 3-17o

The legs are placed in a V above the body and are flexed and extended alternately at the knee to strengthen the adductors at the inside of the thigh. Care should be taken not to open the legs too wide.

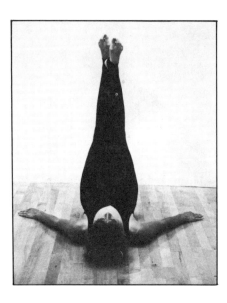

Figure 3-17p

In another strengthening exercise for the adductors, the dancer opens and closes the legs. The legs are alternately crossed with one leg in front and then in back. Care should be taken to open the legs only to a middle range of motion at the hip joint.

During the warm-up, it is typical for beginners to experience some problems with strengthening exercises until they have learned how to position the body properly. In the abdominal curl, for example, it is important to keep the feet firmly on the floor and to curl up and down from the floor one vertebra at a time. A better feeling for the correct performance of the sit-up can be achieved by practicing the curling action up and down from the floor very slowly. Under no circumstances should you place the back down on the floor while it is arched when uncurling from a sit-up (figure 3-18).

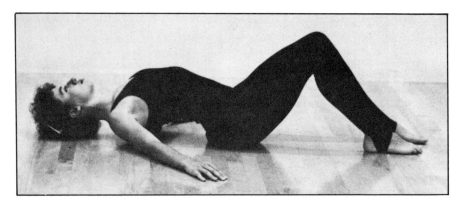

Figure 3-18

In performing an abdominal curl or sit-up, the spine should be lifted off the floor one vertebrae at a time. This process is reversed while curling back down to the floor. Under no circumstances should the back be placed down on the floor in the incorrect position shown above.

The greatest problem with stretching is that of improperly applied energy during the stretch. Bouncing while stretching should be avoided, especially at the beginning of the warm-up. A bouncing stretch causes muscle fibers to tense or contract against the direction in which stretching is taking place.[13] A long holding stretch or a slow, gradual movement into a stretch position are much more beneficial. In addition, the main part of a stretch should be experienced in the middle or the belly of the muscle.

Some individuals have had good results increasing their movement range through a stretching technique known as reciprocal innervation. In this method, you contract the muscle group that is opposite the group of muscles you wish to stretch. The contraction should be maintained forcefully against resistance in the midrange of motion for a particular joint for ten to twenty seconds. Forceful contraction is followed by relaxing the muscles and stretching with added pressure in the opposite direction[14] (Figures 3-19, a-b). It is important that muscles be warmed first before stretching, no matter which form of stretching technique is used.

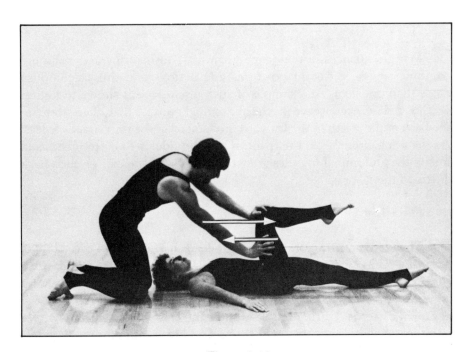

Figure 3-19a

In a reciprocal stretch for the hamstrings, the quadriceps are contracted against resistance in the mid range of motion for the hip joint.

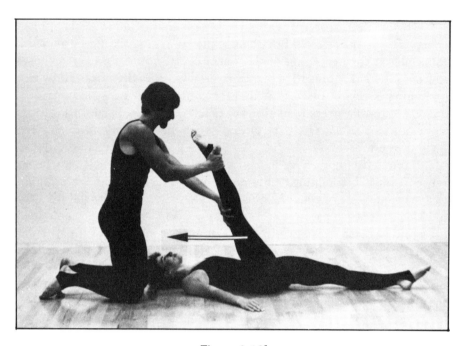

Figure 3-19b
Forceful contraction of the quadriceps is followed by relaxing the muscles, and then stretching the hamstrings.

Many sequences in the dance warm-up (both sitting and standing) combine several different positions and actions and thus accomplish more than one goal. An example of such a sequence is shown in figures 3-20, a-d. This exercise works the abdominal muscles first, then stretches the back and the legs in the forward movement of the torso over the legs. As the arms circle back, the front of the shoulder area is stretched, and finally the abdominal muscles are worked again as the dancer curls back down to the floor.

Standing Warm-Up

The seated portion of the warm-up leads naturally into the standing warm-up. Here, movements for the arms, legs, and feet are emphasized. The torso, shoulders, and head may remain quiet or be moved in combination with actions of the extremities in order to practice more complex patterns. During this section of the class, many teachers prefer to alternate sharp movements of the feet and legs with more continuous actions of the body and arms. The portion of the warm-up performed while standing also helps improve flexibility and strength while attempting to develop body awareness and accuracy at the same time.

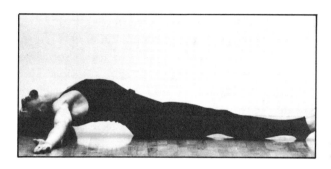

Figure 3-20a
*The above movement
sequence works the
abdominal muscles first,*

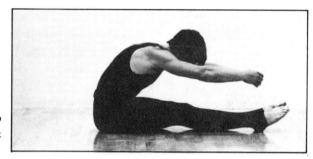

Figure 3-20b
*and then stretches the back
and legs.*

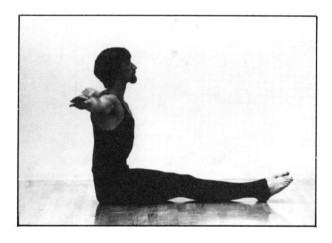

Figure 3-20c
*As the body moves to the
vertical, the arms circle
back to stretch the muscles
at the front of the
shoulders.*

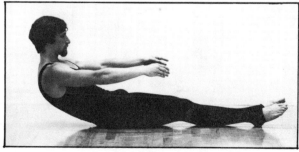

Figure 3-20d
*Finally, the abdominals
are strengthened again as
the body is uncurled to
the floor.*

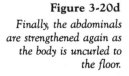

Six basic positions are found in modern dance, although fifth and sixth positions are generally reserved for intermediate students (Figures 3-21, a-i). Figure 3-22 demonstrates where the leg and foot should be placed in second position when performing leg gestures to the side. This forward diagonal placement of the leg should always be used in movements such as pointing, brushing, and lifting of the leg in second and is often referred to as a working second position. On the other hand, the legs and feet are placed more directly to the side of the body when the weight is taken on both feet in second (Figure 3-23).

In addition to the six basic positions, the legs can be turned parallel or inward at the hip joint or outward, as demonstrated in the six basic positions (Figure 3-24). In performing the six positions, the body is kept square. This means that the front of each shoulder and hipbone remains facing forward rather than twisting sideways. When one or both arms are extended to the side, they are held slightly in front of the body, rather than behind the body, to avoid overarching of the back (Figure 3-25). To avoid a hunched shoulder look, the arms are placed lower than the shoulders and are turned outward so that the elbows are hidden from view. Energy should flow from shoulders to fingertips so that there is no sharp break at the wrists (Figure 3-26).

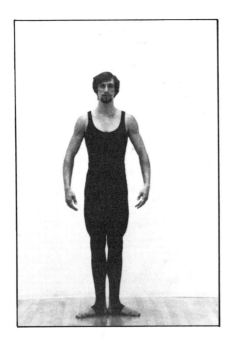

Figure 3-21a
First position.

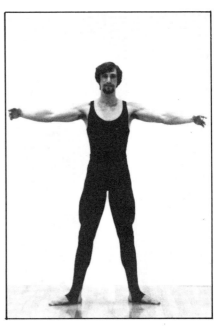

Figure 3-21b
Second position.

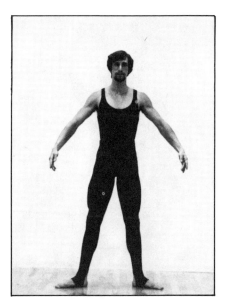

Figure 3-21c

Second position with the arms lower. (Demi-second)

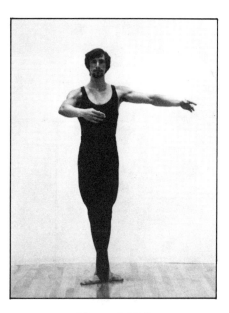

Figure 3-21d

Third position. In this position the heel of the front foot is placed at the instep of the back foot.

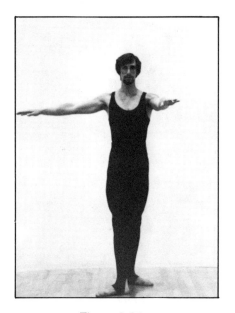

Figure 3-21e

Fourth position. In this position the feet are apart at the distance of one foot length, with the heel of the forward foot in front of the instep of the back foot.

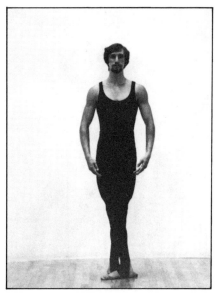

Figure 3-21f

Fifth position with arms low. In this position the heel of the front foot is placed next to the base of the big toe of the back foot.

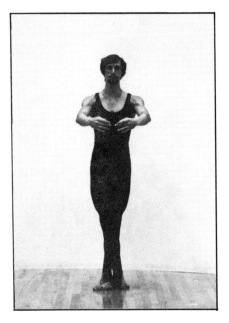

Figure 3-21g
Fifth position, arms at middle level.

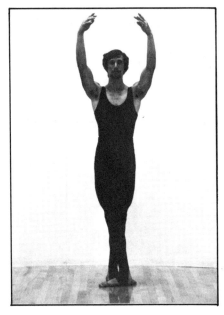

Figure 3-21h
Fifth position, arms high.

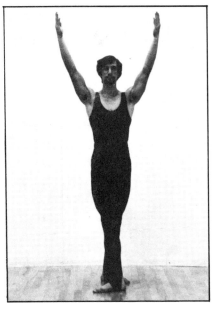

Figure 3-21i
Sixth position. In this position the feet are apart at the distance of one foot length, with the heel of the forward foot in front of the base of the big toe of the back foot.

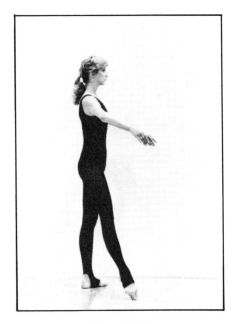

Figure 3-22
Working second position with leg on forward diagonal.

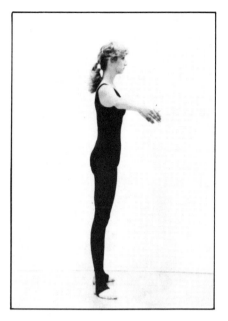

Figure 3-23

When the weight is on both feet, the leg moves more directly to the side in second position.

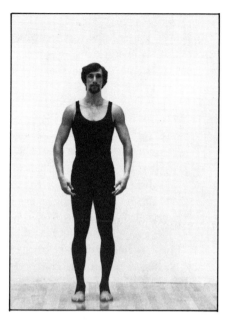

Figure 3-24

Parallel position.

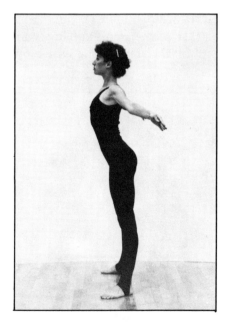

Figure 3-25

Incorrect alignment with the back overarched, and the arms held behind the body.

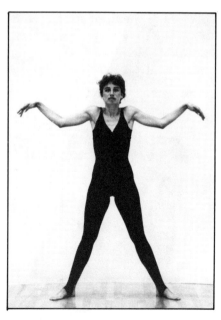

Figure 3-26

Incorrect stance with shoulders too high, and with the energy flow blocked at joints.

Customary positions of the body are similar to those found during the seated part of the warm-up, with the addition of a few more positions possible while standing (Figures 3-27, a-v). The sequence of movements found in the second part of the warm-up is usually as follows:

1. Stretching movement in the center of the body.
2. Plié sequence combining demi, grand plié, and sometimes relevé.
3. Small movements of the legs and feet such as pointing, brushing, circling; exercises in which the ball of the foot is pushed against the floor; or those in which the foot is lifted quickly upward.
4. Larger movements of the leg from the hip joint, including kicking, swinging, or circling.

The plié has been part of the dance warm-up for many years. It dates back to ballet technique that preceded the origins of modern dance. In performing the plié correctly, you must lift the center away from the floor as already discussed (Figure 3-4, a). Second, the head and shoulders must remain above the hips, with the knees over the middle toes when the body is viewed in profile (Figures 3-28, a-b). In a demi plié, the heels are kept on the floor to increase the stretch at the back of the lower leg. In grand plié, the heels come off the floor as the center is lowered downward. During the ascent from a grand plié, the heels should be pressed to the floor so that you move through demi plié (Figures 3-29, a-c). The only exception to this rule is that of the grand plié in second position. Here the heels stay on the floor throughout the entire plié movement.

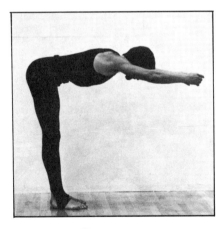

Figure 3-27a

A common position used as part of standing portion of the warm-up. The back should be parallel to the floor.

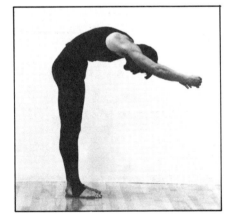

Figure 3-27b

Incorrect with back rounded.

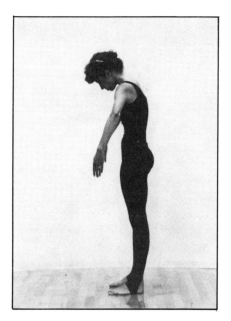

Figure 3-27c
Curving forward from the waist.

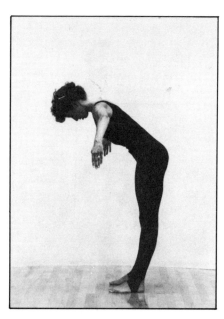

Figure 3-27d
Incorrect performance of curve forward from waist so that hips are flexed instead.

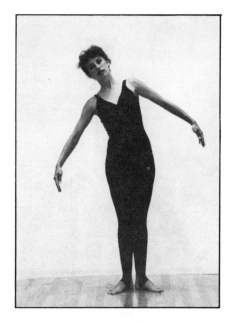

Figure 3-27e
Side curve in spine from waist.

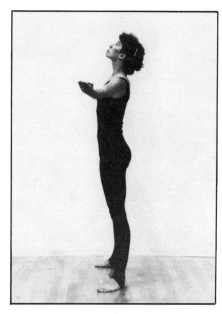

Figure 3-27f
Arching upper back.

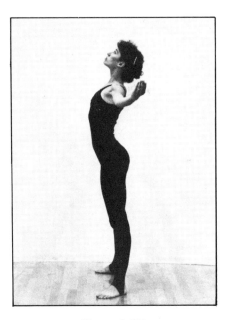

Figure 3-27g

Incorrect upper back arch taken too low in spine.

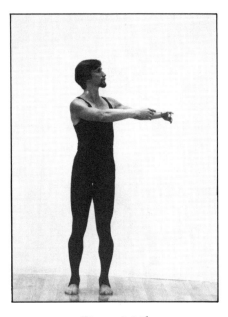

Figure 3-27h

Rotation of the spine. Hips and knees should remain facing forward.

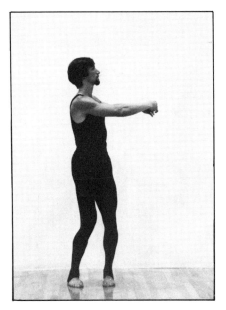

Figure 3-27i

Incorrect rotation in spine so that dancer has hips facing the diagonal. Knees are twisted, and there is a rolling inward on the arch of one foot.

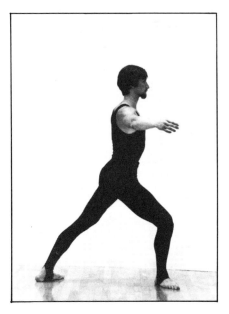

Figure 3-27j

Lunge forward at middle level.

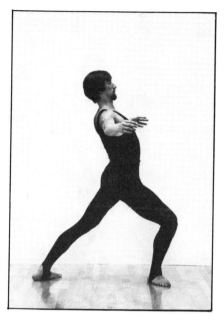

Figure 3-27k

Incorrect forward lunge with head too far back and back overarched.

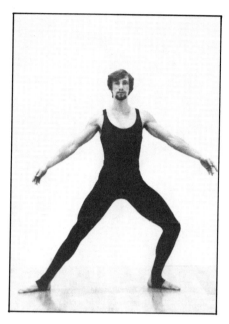

Figure 3-27l
Side lunge.

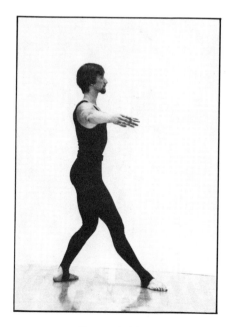

Figure 3-27m
Backward lunge.

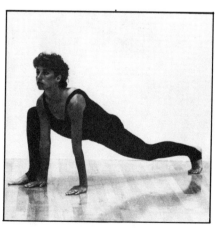

Figure 3-27n
Lunge forward at low level.

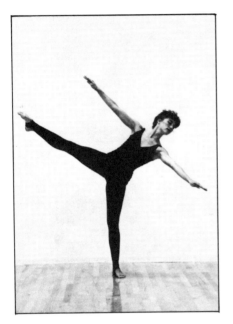

Figure 3-27o
Tilt.

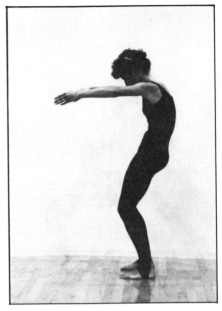

Figure 3-27p
Contraction of center of body in abdominal area.

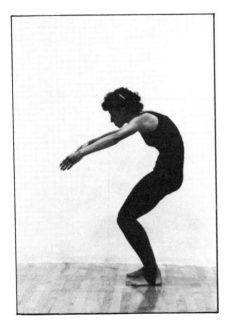

Figure 3-27q
Incorrect contraction with weight dropped and head too far forward.

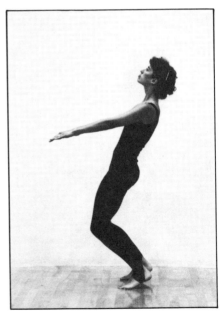

Figure 3-27r
Hinge standing.

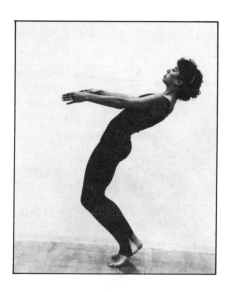

Figure 3-27s
Incorrect hinge with overarched back.

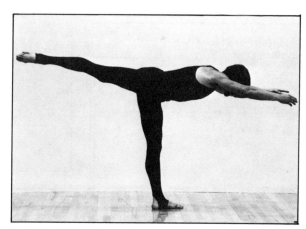

Figure 3-27t
Arabesque parallel to the floor. As straight a line as possible should be maintained from the hands and head to the foot reaching backward.

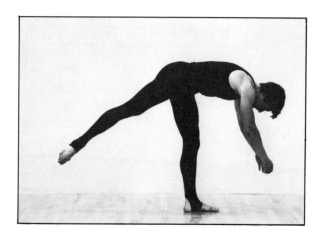

Figure 3-27u
Incorrect arabesque.

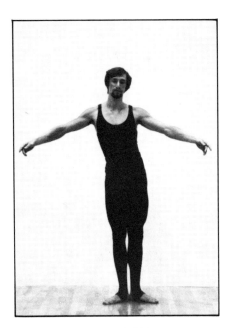

Figure 3-27v
Shift in ribs to side.

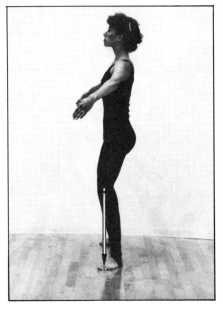

Figure 3-28a
Plié in profile. Knee falls over the middle toe.

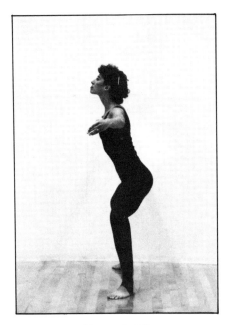

Figure 3-28b
Incorrect plié with head forward and hips too far back.

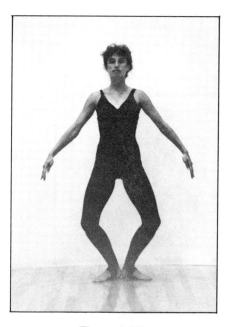

Figure 3-29a

The dancer moves through demi plié at the beginning of grand plié. Note how the heels are placed down on the floor.

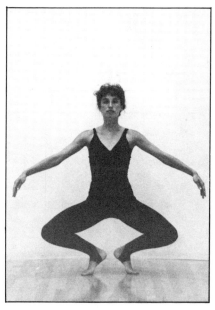

Figure 3-29b

As the dancer moves further into grand plié, the heels gradually come off the floor. The center remains lifted throughout movement sequence.

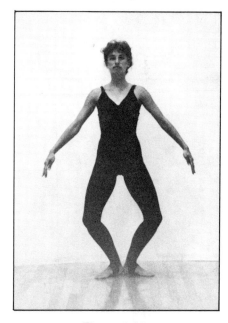

Figure 3-29c

When recovering from grand plié, the dancer again passes through the demi plié position.

Sometimes a relevé, or rising to half toe, is added after recovery from the plié. A relevé is easily accomplished by lifting the center to the ceiling and pressing down through the legs against the floor. Many beginners, however, perform a relevé by lifting the shoulders rather than by lifting the center of gravity. Care should be taken to maintain body alignment throughout a relevé (Figures 3-30, a-c).

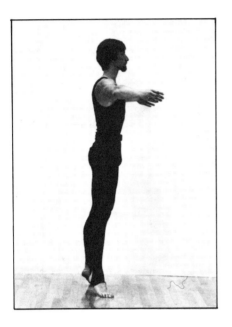

Figure 3-30a
Relevé.

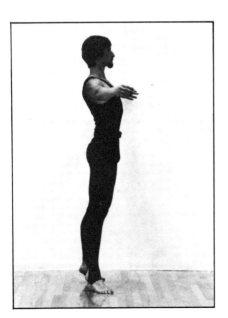

Figure 3-30b
Incorrect relevé with shoulders lifting rather than performing lift in center.

Figure 3-30c
Incorrect relevé with upper body too far back.

Balance is important when doing the small warm-up movements of the feet. To increase stability, position the center above the supporting foot. It is wrong to shift the weight into the hip of the supporting leg or into the working foot (Figure 3-31, a-c). When pointing or brushing the foot, you should also get the energy to the tips of the toes. Otherwise, the

Figure 3-31a

Warm-up movement of foot with center correctly placed above support.

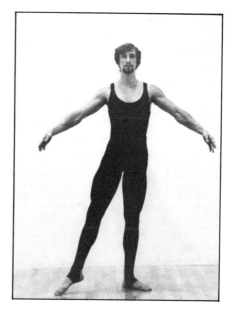

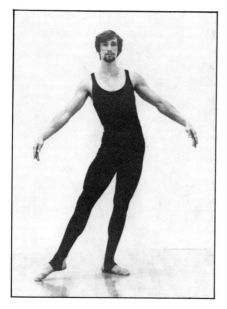

Figure 3-31b

Incorrect with center to the side of supporting foot.

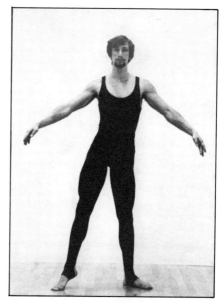

Figure 3-31c

Incorrect with weight shifted to working leg rather than above base.

foot will appear limp or unattractive (Figure 3-32). In brushes performed with a flexed foot, the energy projects from the heel. Other warm-up sequences for the feet are pushing and circling actions (Figures 3-33, a-b and 3-34, a-c). Pushing movements should be performed quickly with a sharp quality.

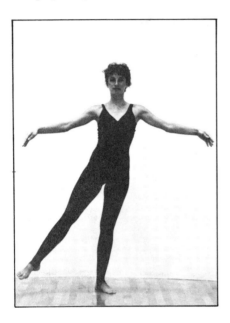

Figure 3-32
Incorrect brush with no energy extended into toes.

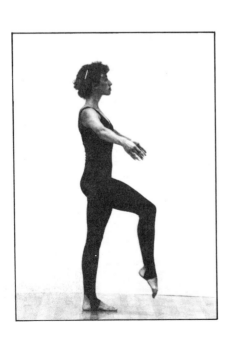

Figure 3-33a
A common warm-up exercise for the ankle and foot.

Figure 3-33b
In this sequence, the foot is pushed sharply off the floor so that the ankle extends with the toes directed toward the floor.

Figure 3-34a

Another warm-up sequence for the feet and ankles involves a circling action of the working leg.

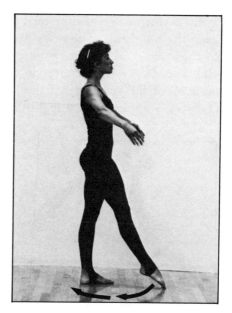

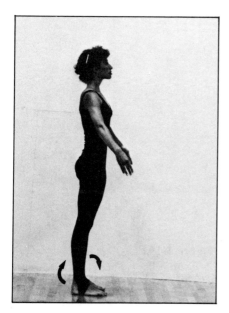

Figure 3-34b

Here the foot has been drawn in toward the supporting foot.

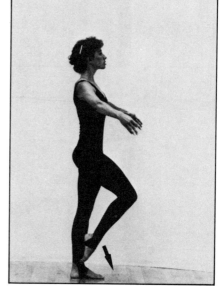

Figure 3-34c

To complete the circling action, the foot is lifted to the ankle and then is moved forward to the original position.

Movements done with the whole leg require even greater balance. Here again, you should locate the center of gravity over the base as the leg is moved. It is also important to keep the center lifted, to project energy out through the toes of the working leg, and to keep the head above the hips. A leg lift done to the side is an illusion, since this movement is really performed on the forward diagonal of working second in order to keep the hip down. The exact placement of this diagonal is determined by the amount of outward rotation that each individual has in the hip. If you would do a leg lift directly to the side, the hip would have to lift because of the structure of the joint, creating a very unattractive line (Figures 3-35, a-b). In a leg lift done to the back, the body must tilt

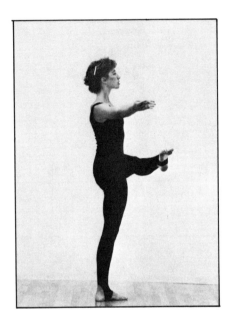

Figure 3-35a
A leg lift performed to the side is actually done on the forward diagonal, or in working second.

Figure 3-35b
Incorrect leg lift side. The dancer has placed her working leg directly to the side of her body, causing her hip to be too high.

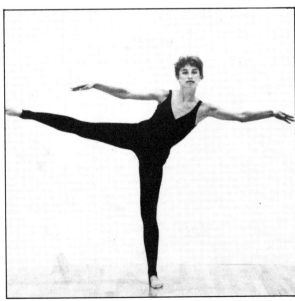

forward somewhat to avoid overarching the lower portion of the spine (figures 3-36, a-b). In a leg swing, the center again is placed right above the base of support. The tendency among beginners, however, is to allow the hips to move in whatever direction the leg is swinging. The working leg also passes through first position with the heel on the floor as it moves from front to back (Figures 3-37, a-d).

Dancing

The remainder of the modern dance class is made up of single locomotor steps or combinations of locomotors that move across the floor or around the dance area depending on how your teacher wishes to use the studio or gymnasium space. Your teacher will choose the locomotor steps to be learned in each lesson. Locomotors commonly used in modern dance are: walk, run, hop, jump, slide, skip, leap, and various types of turns. Generally, some form of sound accompaniment is provided once the locomotor combination is learned so that you can practice the steps with music or rhythmic accompaniment, and get more of the feeling of dancing.

Alignment should be maintained as nearly as possible when performing locomotor steps. In a walk or run, for example, it is very

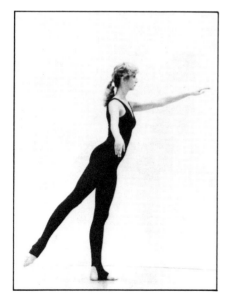

Figure 3-36a
Leg lift to back.

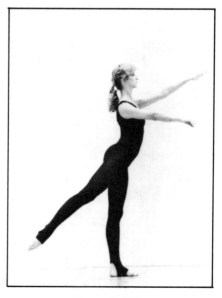

Figure 3-36b
Incorrect leg lift back. Body remains in vertical position causing too much arch in back.

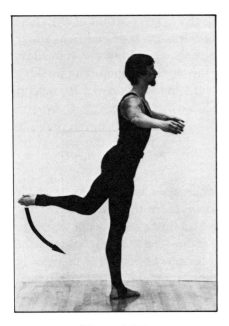

Figure 3-37a

The leg swing begins with the leg behind the body.

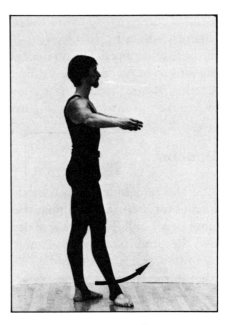

Figure 3-37b

As the leg drops toward the floor, it passes through first position, and then continues forward.

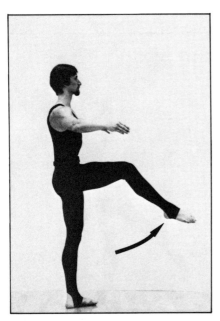

Figure 3-37c

End of forward leg swing.

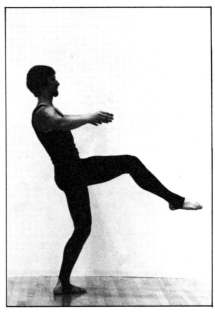

Figure 3-37d

Incorrect forward leg swing. Center is dropped toward floor and the head is behind the hips.

unattractive to lead with the head or to have the hips trailing behind the body (Figures 3-3, a-b). Usually in a walk, the arms swing at a low level forward and back in opposition to the movement of the legs. In a run, the arms are held at your sides, since swinging them projects a frantic, hurried feeling that is distracting to the observer. It is also important in both the walk and run to reach out through the legs, putting the toes down on the floor first. The rest of the foot then rolls down to the floor in a smooth action. The major difference between the walk and the run is not only one of the tempo. In a walk, one foot touches the floor as the other foot leaves the floor, while in a run, there is one point where both feet are off the ground.[15]

The hop and jump are very similar except that in a hop you land on one foot, and in a jump you land on two feet.[16] Upon landing, the foot rolls to the floor — toe, ball, heel — and the knees bend to cushion the landing (Figures 3-38, a-c). It is incorrect to perform a series of jumps without getting the heels on the floor between each jump, and you should try not to roll in on the inner border of the foot upon landing (Figure 3-39). Getting the heels down also stretches out the back of the lower leg and saves this part of the body from possible injury. Throughout the hop or jump, the body maintains alignment, and the arms are kept alongside the body so that they do not make distracting movements (Figure 3-40). The legs are straight when the dancer is in the air, and the ankles are extended with pointed toes (Figures 3-41, a-b).

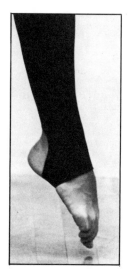
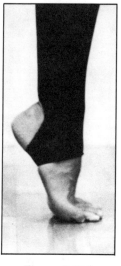
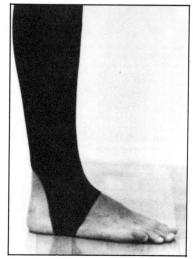

Figure 3-38a
The toes touch first, as the foot moves back to the floor.

Figure 3-38b
Next the ball of the foot, and then the heel come down.

Figure 3-38c

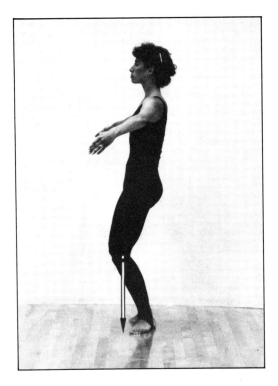

Figure 3-39
Incorrect placement during a landing from a jump. The knees are too far forward, and the feet are rolled inward on the arches.

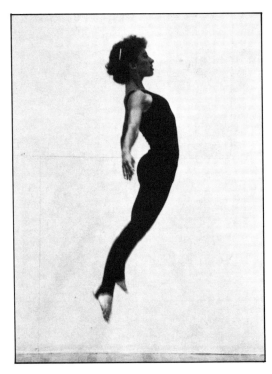

Figure 3-40
Incorrect alignment during jump.

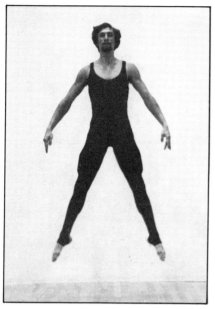

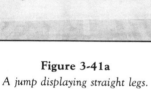

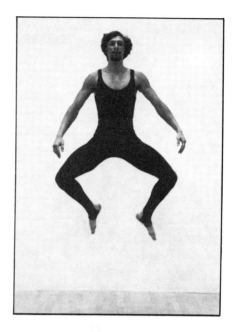

Figure 3-41a
A jump displaying straight legs.

Figure 3-41b
Incorrect jump with legs relaxed.

In a slide, a gliding step is taken to the side, then a second step is taken to close the feet in a cutting action as the body is propelled into the air.[17] The feet actually move through first and second positions in a slide. When the body is in the air, the legs are again straight, as they are in a jump (Figures 3-42, a-d). At times, various arm movements are combined with the sliding steps.

A skip is actually a step and a hop combined.[18] The body is propelled into the air while one leg remains straight and underneath the body. The other leg is lifted with a bent knee in front of the body, or at the side on the diagonal if a skip is being performed in a side direction. Alignment is maintained throughout the movement with the shoulders above the hips, and the landing is on the take-off leg without a change of weight (Figures 3-43, a-e). Sometimes, the skip is combined with one or two preparatory steps between each skipping movement.

A leap changes weight upon landing. During the leap, the center of gravity traces an arc in space, both feet are off the floor, and the body is suspended midair.[19] A common problem in a leap is to bicycle the legs when you are in the air. To avoid this error, straighten the back leg to push against the floor, and reach forward through the front leg so that both legs are straight and extended out from your center in opposite

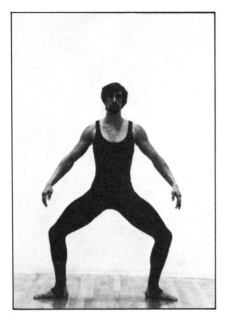

Figure 3-42a
The slide begins with a plié.

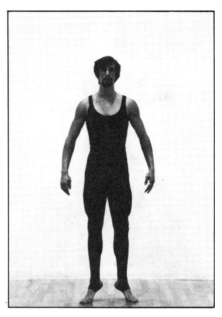

Figure 3-42b
The dancer then brings the legs together and pushes into the air.

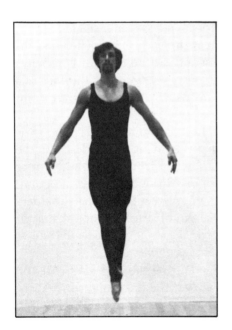

Figure 3-42c

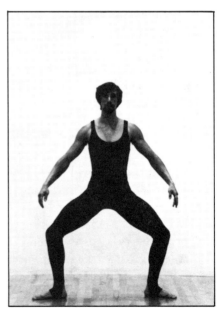

Figure 3-42d
The slide ends in plié to cushion the landing.

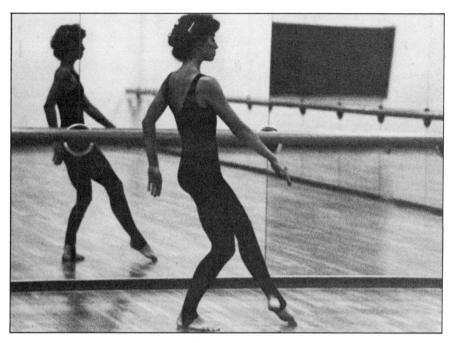

Figure 3-43a
The dancer steps forward to prepare for the skip,

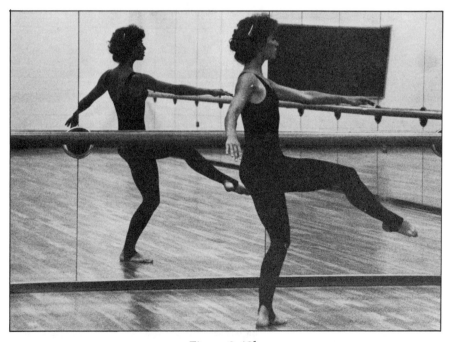

Figure 3-43b

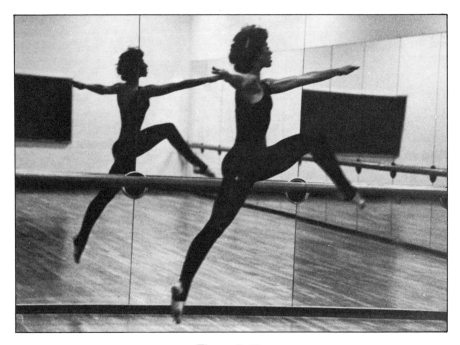

Figure 3-43c
pushes into the air, and

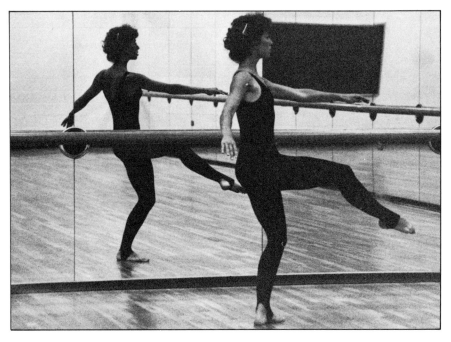

Figure 3-43d
lands on the same leg which she used to propel her body into the air.

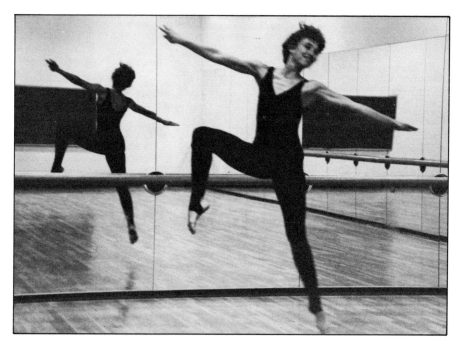

Figure 3-43e
A skip to the side.

directions at the highest point in the leap. The plié and rolling action of the lead leg and foot cushion the landing (Figures 3-44, a-c).

Turns can also be considered locomotor movements when they travel in space. In performing a turn, it is important to keep the body aligned. Leaning in one direction or another, or breaking the body line at the neck or the hips, will cause you to fall in whatever direction you have the most weight (Figures 3-45, a-c). In many turns, it is appropriate to use the head to help perform the turn. This action of the head is called whipping or spotting and helps you keep your balance. You will not get dizzy while turning if you learn to spot correctly. In spotting, the face and eyes are fixed on one point at eye level off in the direction toward which you are turning. As you start to turn, the head and eyes remain fixed on the orientation point. Finally, when the turn is half finished, as it is impossible to keep the head in its fixed position, you whip the head around to allow you to immediately fixate on the orientation point again.[20] Spotting can be practiced by fixing the eyes in one place, then taking tiny turning steps until a full rotation is accomplished. Halfway through the series of small turning steps, the head is whipped around. Spotting with the head is used in many types of modern dance turns. In

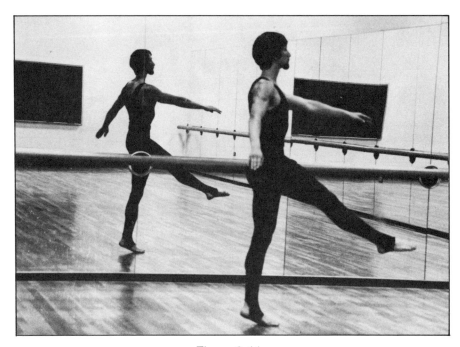

Figure 3-44a
In preparing to leap the dancer extends the lead leg,

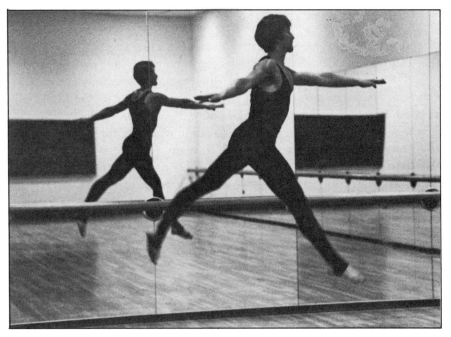

Figure 3-44b
pushes off with back leg, and

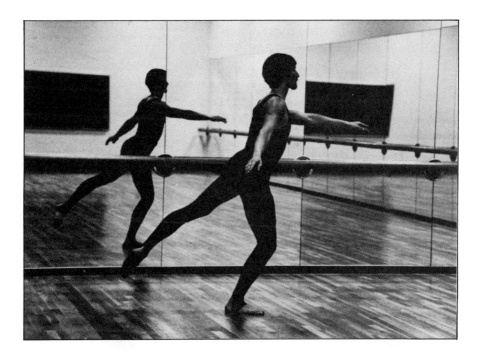

Figure 3-44c
lands in demi plié on the lead leg. During the leap, the center of the body traces an arc in the space.

other kinds of modern dance turns, particularly those done in intermediate and advanced level classes, such a whipping action is not possible, since the body is placed in other than a vertical position and the focus is on the ceiling or floor.

Your teacher will provide you with many combinations of the different locomotor steps throughout your class. Try to see which locomotors are being presented when the combination is demonstrated.

Warm-Down

It is important to take time to slow down gradually at the conclusion of your dance class. Some slow movements and stretches will usually be provided in the center floor area for this purpose. The warm-down takes about five to ten minutes. At the end of the warm-down, the heart rate should be back to normal.

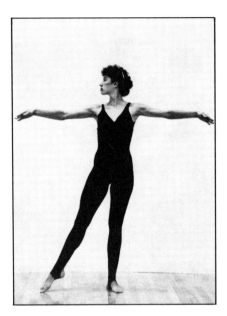

Figure 3-45a

The dancer prepares to turn by looking to the side.

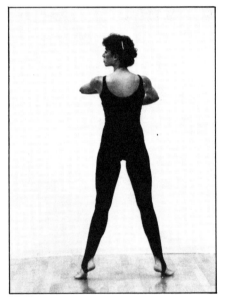

Figure 3-45b

As the dancer continues to turn, the focus remains in the original direction.

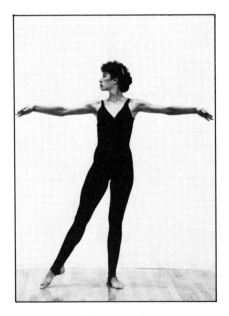

Figure 3-45c

Finally, when focus can no longer be maintained, the head whips around to look in the original direction again.

Tips

In attempting to learn a movement combination, try to see the overall framework of the pattern first. Observe the starting point of the combination — where it goes and how it concludes. Doing the pattern with only the body and legs, then adding the arms and head later, may also help.

Counting may help you initially in learning sequences of movement, but do not get overly involved in counting. An easier method of understanding rhythmic patterning is to sense where the movement is faster than the underlying basic beat, where it is slower, and where you are dancing on the beat of the accompaniment. [21]Figure 3-46 is a diagram of the pattern created over the basic beat by several different locomotor steps.

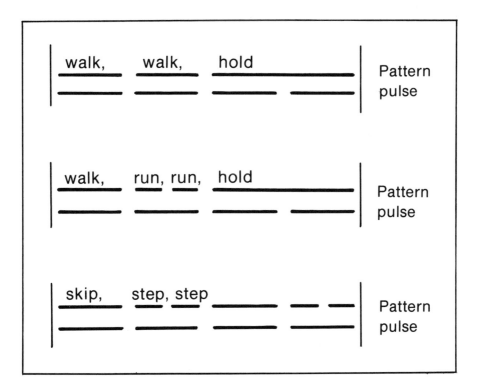

Figure 3-46
The top line in each drawing indicates the pattern created by the locomotor steps.

When you have an understanding of the basic structure of a movement pattern, try to have fun with it. If you make a mistake, pick up the movement and try again. Do not be negative and waste time by scolding yourself for making errors. Get involved in your actions; relax and concentrate on what they really feel like.[22] Put your energy behind the action and dance, rather than marking time. In other words, try to perform the movements. Make the energy project beyond your own body so that there is a sense of continuity in your actions, not a feeling of simply going from one position to the next. The above suggestions should apply to learning both center floor and locomotor sequences.

Creative Work

Your teacher may decide to include some creative experiences in your beginning modern dance class. This creative work may be in the form of improvisation or short pieces of choreography known as dance studies. In either instance, some kind of framework will be provided within which the creative movement is to be developed.

In the case of improvisational work, try to relate to the suggestions given by the instructor and let your body start moving. Be relaxed, and let yourself respond and allow your energies to flow from the motivation.[23] Relate to your teacher's suggestions in as many ways as you can think of, using the full movement potential for each part of your body. Play with the movements, allowing one movement to lead you into the next series of actions. Try not to worry about the other people in the class, but concentrate on yourself and on how you really feel in relation to the suggestions given by the teacher.

Some examples of improvisational experiences follow. Find a partner and decide who is to be leader. Let one person mirror the movements of the other. As you move, see how many different ways you can move various body parts. Try changing levels. Another improvisational experience might be to move around the room, stopping in different body shapes when the accompaniment stops. When you stop, take your shape over to the person nearest to you and continue to move, relating your body shapes to each other.

In dance composition or choreography, movement is found through improvisation, and it is then set into a structured dance.[24] The entire dance or study is made up of many short pieces of movement known as phrases. A simple dance, for example, could be created by using a long word or series of words as the starting point. Your teacher might ask you to say the word or words in different ways, supplying movement phrases that you feel have the same quality as the various intonations of the word.

Your teacher will probably have many different ways of improvising and doing creative work.

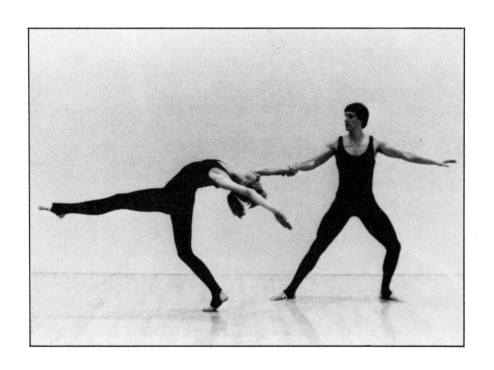

CHAPTER 4

The Mind

Dance is very physical, but the mind is also important in learning to dance and can aid physical learning.

Concentration

When beginning a dance class, it is important to be present with both your body and mind. You cannot come to class having your mind preoccupied with other affairs. In other words, the mind and body need to work together. When movements are demonstrated, you should experience them totally with both mind and body.

Concentration can be increased through the use of relaxation exercises done before class. One way of relaxing is to sit or lie quietly and bring all your energies back to yourself; emphasize your breathing and its rhythm. Noted kinesiologist Lulu Swiegard recommended what she called the constructive rest position for purposes of relaxation (Figure 4-1).[1] The point here is to attempt to release tension in the back so that it can relax into the floor, and to support the limbs in a way that does not require muscular tension.

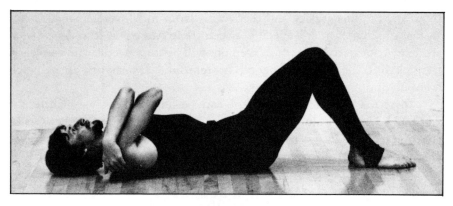

Figure 4-1
Constructive rest position with feet flat on the floor, legs parallel and with the arms draped over the chest.

The use of various images can aid relaxation and concentration. Here it is important to try to visualize the image in your mind, then transfer the basic feeling of that image to your body. The following images have been found to facilitate relaxation: (1) a floating feather; (2) lying on a very comfortable bed; (3) the feeling of the whole body floating; and (4) lying on a beach on a warm summer day.

Seeing Movement

Movement is a part of our daily life but is often overlooked and taken for granted. In other words, we do not really see human movement because it has become utilitarian for most of us. In dance, movement is the media of the art and must be experienced in all of its variety.

One way of looking at movement is in terms of an anatomical analysis. Thus, you could see when a flexion, extension, rotation, abduction, or adduction was occurring as a dance combination was being demonstrated. It would also be important to see how each of these movements connected with and flowed into the next.

Movement is made up of space, shape, energy, and time, which are known as its elements. We can use an understanding of these elements to help in perceiving movement. Space, for example, includes the aspects of level, direction, and size, while shape provides sculptural forms. Energy causes movements that can be sustained (slow and continuous), percussive (direct and explosive), or vibratory (shaking and trembling). Additional energy qualities are to be suspended as in a balance or a leap, to collapse by releasing a part or all of the body into gravity, or to swing by dropping into gravity and recovering from it. Movement tempo can be fast or slow or at any speed between these two opposites. As a dance student, your perception of movement will be improved if you can learn to pick out the spacial, energy, or temporal framework in a dance combination.

In terms of space, movement can be analyzed in many different ways. (1) You might look at the pathway traced by various body parts in space (Figure 4-2), or the various planes in which movements travel (Figure 4-3). (2) The pattern traced on the floor is another important aspect of a combination. (3) Note how level changes take place. (4) There are eight basic directions generally used in dance class (Figure 4-4).[2] Learn to see in which direction movement travels, where arms and legs are placed in relation to the body, and whether turns are performed outward or inward from the body's midline.

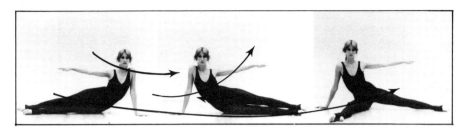

Figure 4-2

Pathways created by different parts of the body as these body parts are moved through space.

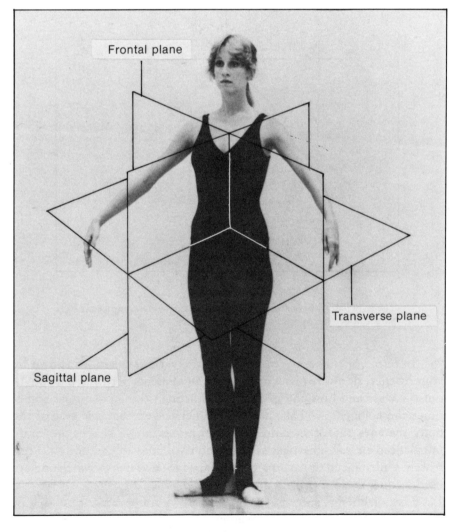

Figure 4-3

Some of the planes in space in which movement can occur.

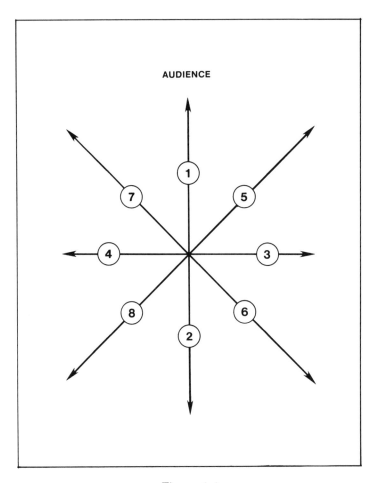

Figure 4-4

The eight basic directions in which the body can move or in which the body parts can be extended.

In terms of shape, try to duplicate the various positions shown by your teacher. Be aware of such shapes in movements performed throughout the class and how the body moves through these positions. Sometimes these shapes are balanced or symmetrical so that one side of the body matches the other side. At other times, these shapes are more unbalanced or asymmetrical so that the two sides of the body do not match. Unbalanced or asymmetrical shapes are exciting to watch and are used frequently in modern dance (Figure 3-11).

Use of energy, likewise, creates its own framework. Impulses of energy are applied to initiate movement; they continue, and finally reach a conclusion. You should be able to pick up on the variation in energy quality that occurs during a combination.

The varying tempo of movements in a combination can also be analyzed. Most pieces of movement have a steady underlying pulse beat, which is the same as the pulse beat in the accompaniment. Develop an awareness of this beat. Usually, your teacher will clap or count on this pulse. Next, note how movement tends to go with the basic beat at times, while at other times, it is faster or slower than the pulse. Try to see what kinds of patterns these changes in speed of movement produce. Chanting the various rhythmic patterns to yourself as you perform the combination may be helpful.

The elements of movement — space, shape, energy, and time — also have varying feeling qualities associated with them. A large use of space is very expansive and creates a more joyful feeling, whereas a small movement is more reserved or quiet. Quick movement is exciting, while slow movement can be calm or even boring in its expression. Vibratory use of energy is tense and nervous; percussive energy can be daring or angry; and swinging movement is very relaxing and playful. Furthermore, suspended movement can take your breath away as it hovers in midair, and a collapse has an exhausting feeling about it. Try to sense the feeling qualities of each movement, since this can make doing these actions a more exciting experience, and can also help you correct performance problems.

Another important factor in learning movements is to understand weight placement. You need to notice which foot bears the weight at the beginning of a combination. Differentiate between placing weight on one or two feet, be ready for quick changes of weight, and remember that weight is not placed on the foot performing gestures such as pointing or brushing.

Visualizing

Use of mental imagery or pictures can improve your dance ability. Such imagery is particularly useful for increasing understanding of correct alignment. Some images that you can try are to see your neck growing longer so that you feel yourself growing taller.[3] Thinking of your ribs as narrowing at the front of your body and the pelvis as broadening across the back, or imagining your spine as lengthening downward, can also be helpful in finding proper alignment.[4] Another image used to correct alignment is that of energy or water streaming up through the center of the body and washing down the outsides.[5]

Images are also used to improve performance of various dance movements, For example, to help with the lengthening feeling needed in a leg lift, imagine energy streaming out through your toes. The slightly rounded arms in second position can be likened to the mental picture of holding a very large beach ball in your arms.[6]

Listen carefully to the different mental pictures and cues that your dance teacher uses. Concentrate and try to experience them in your own body, since your instructor will probably have many creative and helpful images of his/her own.

Using Your Senses

Your teacher will probably use various methods to explain the correct way of doing a movement. Some cues will be more visual, some verbal, and others will be kinesthetic in origin. Relate first to the visual demonstration, and try to act on your impressions of the shapes and lines that you see as part of the actions.[7] Second, listen carefully to verbal descriptions, since your teacher's words are meant to supplement the visual.[8] Finally, try to find what you saw and heard in your own body. At times, you might ask your teacher to help position or move your body so that you can get the right feeling of a movement.[9] As you progress in your study of dance, begin to build up a collection of your own muscular feelings that you can recall when performing the many different movements of modern dance.

Adding It Up

Technique, improvisation, and composition are all important parts of modern dance. Most beginning classes deal with technique and perhaps some improvisation to give students a taste of creative work. All three of these areas, however, are related. Technique builds movement skill so that you have increased body control. With good technique, improvisation and composition work are not as limited, since you have a wider range of movement within your grasp.[10] Improvisation also leads into composition, because it is the method by which you experiment and find movements for a choreography.[11]

Modern dance has changed since its beginnings. Like any art form, it has varied in response to trends and ideas prevalent during different times. In the 1940-1950 period, it was the style to choreograph dances that told a story and projected meaning to the audience. Many of Martha Graham's works from this era, for instance, were dance dramas — a form of dance that is known as literal choreography today.[12]

By the 1960s, dancers had become less concerned with telling stories. Dances still needed to be based on some intent, but the finished choreography was much more abstract in nature. Only the essence or basic feeling associated with the original motivation needed to come across to the audience.

The 1970s brought even less concern for projection of meaning to those viewing a dance. This was the period of experimentation in which movement was used in a composition for its own sake, not for the purpose of conveying a feeling or idea to those watching. These new choreographies were called nonliteral.[13] Modern dancers Merce Cunningham and Alwin Nikolais became masters of this choreographic method, although their particular dance styles differ.

When you go to a dance concert, be open to the style and meaning of each dance. Do not expect all choreography to have a message, and enjoy each dance for what it is in its own right. Other ideas that you can try to experience when viewing a dance concert are as follows:

1. See the overall form of the dance. Try to connect the beginning, middle, and end of a composition through time, being aware of how a dance begins and where it goes.[14]

2. Try to understand the use of the stage space. Watch the dancers travel around the stage, and note relationships between dancers, seeing the dance as a whole, like a picture within the frame of the prosenium arch, rather than by viewing many separate and unrelated figures on stage. It is also important to realize that figures on stage tend to have a more or less powerful image depending on where they are placed onstage.[15] Center stage, for example, attracts the most attention.

3. Notice movement motifs. As you view a dance, you will see certain movements or phrases repeated. Try to understand how the choreographer has varied these phrases and alternated them between the different performers.

4. Attempt to analyze the choreographer's use of space, shape, energy, and time. Gradually, you should become aware of how the elements of movement have been manipulated throughout a dance to contribute to the overall style or emotional effect. Try to see how changes in space, shape, energy, and time affect the feeling or feelings projected from a work.

5. Learn to differentiate one dance style from another. A dance may be lyric, which is a smooth, graceful style somewhat similar to the use of energy in classical ballet. The dance might also be choreographed in a jazz style with sensuous movements and syncopated rhythms like those incorporated in jazz music, or it could be abstract, emphasizing shapes and lines like those in an abstract painting. Choreographies, which heighten the bizarre or

juxtapose and relate the unusual, can project a comical effect and have become popular in recent years.

6. Try to appreciate how the choreographer has used the music. The dance and music should have a complementary relationship rather than one dominating the other.

7. The costumes and lighting design should also complement the dance. Notice if this happens, or if costumes and lighting actually detract from your experiencing the choreography.

NOTES

Chapter 1

1. Sorrell, Walter, *Dance in Its Time* (Garden City, N.Y.: Anchor Press/ Doubleday, 1981), p. 304.
2. Ibid.
3. Maynard, Olga, *American Modern Dancers* (Boston: Little, Brown and Co., 1965), p. 39.
4. Kraus, Richard and Chapman, Sarah, *History of the Dance in Art and Education*, 2nd ed. (Englewood Cliffs, N.J.: Prentice-Hall, Inc., 1981), p. 126.
5. McDonagh, Don, *Don McDonagh's Complete Guide to Modern Dance* (New York: Popular Library, 1977), p. 32.
6. Maynard, p. 67.
7. Sorell, Walter, *The Dance Has Many Faces* (Cleveland: The World Publishing Co., 1951), p. 33.
8. Maynard, p. 82.
9. Kraus and Chapman, p. 130.
10. Sorell, *The Dance Has Many Faces*, p. 130.
11. Ibid.
12. Ibid., pp. 130-131.
13. Maynard, p. 111.
14. McDonagh, p. 74.
15. Kraus and Chapman, p. 134.
16. Maynard, p. 134.
17. McDonagh, p. 113.
18. Maynard, pp. 136-137.
19. Penrod, James and Plastino, Janice Gudde, *The Dancer Prepares*, 2nd ed. (Palo Alto, California: Mayfield Publishing Co., 1980), p. 51.
20. Kraus and Chapman, p. 141.
21. Maynard, p. 141.
22. Ibid.
23. Ibid., p. 142.
24. Ibid., p. 144.
25. Ibid., p. 258.

Chapter 2

1. Hinson, Marilyn, *Kinesiology* (Dubuque, Iowa: Wm. C. Brown Co., 1977), p. 10.
2. Barham, Jerry N., *Mechanical Kinesiology* (St. Louis: The C. V. Mosby Co., 1978), p. 85.
3. Hinson, p. 12.
4. Ibid.
5. Ibid., p. 15.
6. Sweigard, Lulu E., *Human Movement Potential* (New York: Dodd, Mead and Co., 1974), p. 13.
7. Arnheim, Daniel D., *Dance Injuries*, 2nd ed. (St. Louis: The C. V. Mosby Co., 1980), p. 132.
8. Hinson, p. 26.
9. Barham, p. 74.
10. Hinson, p. 7.
11. Barham, p. 74.
12. Ibid.
13. Ibid.
14. Ibid., p. 78.
15. Ibid., p. 79.
16. Fitt, Sally, *Principles of Kinesiology for Teachers of Dance*, class notes, University of Utah, summer 1982.
17. Ibid.
18. Ibid.
19. Penrod, James and Plastino, Janice Gudde, *The Dancer Prepares*, 2nd ed. (Palo Alto, California: Mayfield Publishing Co., 1980), p. 46.
20. Vincent, L. M., M.D., *The Dancer's Book of Health* (Kansas City: Sheed, Andrews and McMeel, Inc., 1978), p. 134.
21. Cooper, Kenneth, M.D., *The Aerobics Way* (New York: Bantam Books, 1977), pp. 142-143.
22. Arnheim, p. 187.
23. Vincent, p. 33.
24. Arnheim, p. 185.
25. Ibid., p. 204.
26. Vincent, p. 34.
27. Arnheim, p. 207.
28. Vincent, p. 35.
29. Ibid., p. 57.
30. Ibid., p. 63.

Chapter 3

1. Hawkins, Alma, *Creating through Dance* (Englewood Cliffs, N.J.: Prentice-Hall, Inc., 1964), p. 66.
2. Penrod, James and Plastino, Janice Gudde, *The Dancer Prepares*, 2nd ed. (Palo Alto, California: Mayfield Publishing Co., 1980), p. 21.
3. Hinson, Marilyn, *Kinesiology* (Dubuque, Iowa: Wm. C. Brown Co., 1977), p. 17.
4. Ibid., p. 230.
5. Ibid., p. 228.
6. Ibid., p. 229.
7. Hawkins, p. 70.
8. Fitt, Sally, *Principles of Kinesiology for Teachers of Dance*, class notes, University of Utah, summer 1982.
9. Hawkins, pp. 78-79.
10. Ibid., p. 79.
11. Ibid., pp. 79-80.
12. Ibid., p. 80.
13. Arnheim, Daniel D., *Dance Injuries*, 2nd ed. (St. Louis: The C. V. Mosby Co., 1980), p. 81.
14. Fitt, class notes.
15. Hayes, Elizabeth R., *An Introduction to the Teaching of Dance* (New York: The Ronald Press Co., 1964), pp. 48-49.
16. Lockhart, Aileene S., *Modern Dance, Building and Teaching Lessons*, 6th ed. (Dubuque, Iowa: Wm. C. Brown Co., 1982), pp. 72-73.
17. Ibid., pp. 71-72.
18. Hayes, p. 47.
19. Lockhart, p. 74.
20. Ibid., p. 82.
21. Hawkins, pp. 57-58.
22. Gallwey, Timothy and Kriegel, Bob, *Inner Skiing* (New York: Random House, 1977), p. 41.
23. Hawkins, p. 22.
24. Ibid., p. 28.

Chapter 4

1. Sweigard, Lulu E., *Human Movement Potential* (New York: Dodd, Mead and Co., 1974), pp. 215-216.
2. Grant, Gail, *Technical Manual and Dictionary of Classical Ballet*, 2nd ed. (New York: Dover Publications, Inc., 1967), p. 113.
3. Sweigard, p. 249.
4. Ibid., pp. 237-241.
5. Dowd, Irene, *Alignment of the Axial Skeleton*, class notes, Naropa Institute, Boulder, Colorado, summer 1981.
6. Kirby, Joel, *Modern Dance Technique*, class notes, Repertory Dance Theater, University of Utah, summer 1982.
7. Genoff, Karen, "Better Movement Perception for the Beginning Dance Student," *Colorado Journal of Health, Physical Education, Recreation and Dance*, winter 1983, p. 10.
8. Ibid.
9. Ibid.
10. Hawkins, Alma, *Creating through Dance* (Englewood Cliffs, N.J.: Prentice-Hall, Inc., 1964), p. 18.
11. Ibid., p. 28.
12. Turner, Margery J., *Approaches to Nonliteral Choreography* (Pittsburgh: University of Pittsburgh Press, 1971), p. 23.
13. Ibid.
14. Hawkins, p. 92.
15. Ellfeldt, Lois, *A Primer for Choreographers* (Palo Alto, California: National Press Books, 1967), p. 9.

ABOUT THE AUTHORS

Sandra Cerny Minton is program coordinator for dance at the University of Northern Colorado. She has a M.A. in dance from U.C.L.A., and a Ph.D. in Dance and Related Arts from Texas Women's University. Sandra has been teaching modern dance at the college level for sixteen years, and throughout this time she has studied with many dance professionals.

Karen Genoff is a dance instructor at the University of Northern Colorado. She received her M.Ed. degree in Dance from Colorado State University. Karen has studied dance from many professionals, including Alwin Nikolais, Murray Louis, Hanya Holm, and Bill Evans.